LITERATURE LINKS FOR NUTRITION AND HEALTH

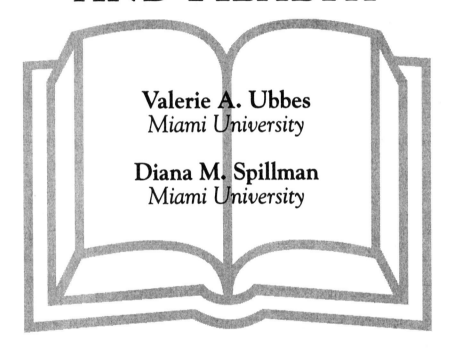

Valerie A. Ubbes
Miami University

Diana M. Spillman
Miami University

D1716444

Allyn and Bacon
Boston London Toronto Sydney Tokyo Singapore

The text font is 12-36 point Times New Roman and 18 point Vivaldi.
Desktop publishing by Valerie A. Ubbes, 1996.

This project was funded in part by the Nutrition Education and Training (NET) Program
(PL102-142) of USDA and the Ohio Department of Education. This program is available
to all individuals regardless of race, color, national origin, age, sex, or handicap. Persons
who believe they have been denied equal opportunity for participation may write to the
Secretary of Agriculture, Washington, DC 20250.

Clip Art used is reproduced from Microsoft Publisher 97. Copyright © Microsoft
Corporation. Used by permission.

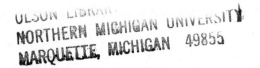

For all children,
especially my children, Allegra and Joshua,
with a special tribute to Bill,
my forever friend and partner.

-VAU

For those who strive to teach, and
those who strive to learn
nutrition.

- DMS

Abbreviated Contents

Unit Contents

Preface (and Acknowledgements)

Preface

Welcome to *Literature Links for Nutrition and Health*. The purpose of this book is to provide elementary teachers and teacher preparation faculty with an integrated curriculum model for teaching nutrition and health to elementary children. Children's literature is used as the medium for teaching and learning about the categorical health topic of nutrition. Through a careful selection process, we have identified 227 picture books for teaching four thematic units: Building the Food Pyramid for grades 1, 2, and 3; Let's Make a Meal for grades 1, 2, and 3; Cycle of Life for grade 2; and World of People for grade 3. You may already read some of these picture books in your classrooms, but perhaps you haven't used them before to teach health-related topics, concepts, and skills.

Literature-Based Lesson Plans for Developing Health-Related Skills

Literature Links for Nutrition and Health shows you how to extend the storylines of picture books for improving the health status of children and youth in your class. We offer you 28 literature-based lesson plans for engaging children in solo, small group, and whole-class activities around 12 focused themes. The lessons help children to use decision making, communication, and goal setting skills in the context of health, nutrition, and eating behaviors. Having up-to-date content knowledge is important and useful. However, using that knowledge to make informed decisions about what to eat, when to eat, with whom, and why to eat are the ultimate learning goals for this curriculum. Four thematic units involve students in participation, application, and performance. Learners will practice, rehearse, and apply health-related skills in various contexts throughout the curriculum.

Integrated Curriculum Model for Promoting Health-Related Concepts

This book links two disciplines, health education and language arts, into an integrated curriculum model, grades 1-3. We acknowledge that nutrition is one of many content areas in comprehensive school health education as outlined in the National Health Education Standards (Joint Committee, 1995, p 12). Because health education often competes for time in a crowded academic curriculum, the lessons in this book make connections across the curriculum from the two featured disciplines, health education and language arts, to six other academic subjects of science, social studies, mathematics, physical education, art, and music. We believe that curriculum design should not compromise the rigor of a discipline for the sake of integration. However, if the critical concepts of a discipline have been identified, then integrated curriculum models can advance and supplement the total curriculum. For example, we draw upon concepts of variety, moderation, energy, time, patterns, age, culture, behavior, and prevention as organizers for our health education units. Concepts are known to bridge disciplines by giving learners a mental schema for building understanding from subject to subject. Conceptual themes are also known to promote higher-level thinking (Erickson, 1999). We believe that both topics and concepts form the basis for sound curriculum design. However, topical units of study are often overused, leading to a simple recall of facts and less understanding.

Content Knowledge Organized by National Nutrition & Health Models
This book is the first *integrated* curriculum model to use the National Health Education Standards (Joint Committee, 1995) as a framework for what students will know and be able to do about their health and well-being in nutrition. The National Health Education Standards guide preK-12 teachers in their decisions about what health-related content and skills they will teach as learner outcomes. All of our literature-based lessons are compared against a checklist of the National Health Education Standards at the beginning of each unit. Unit content is also organized by the Food Guide Pyramid and the Dietary Guidelines for Americans (U.S. Department of Agriculture, 1995). These content decisions ensure that the rigor and contributions of nutrition and health education are sustained from lesson to lesson. This also affords teachers the luxury of extending their own content knowledge in nutrition while in the process of teaching the curriculum -- which may in turn help to enhance their own health and wellbeing during the dynamic interplay of teaching and learning. Because *Literature Links for Nutrition and Health* encourages classroom teachers, food service professionals, parents, caregivers, and other school professionals to collaborate for the health and wellbeing of children, the Coordinated School Health Program (Marx & Wooley, 1998) serves as a useful model for interprofessional approaches during the implementation of the curriculum. Although one teacher in one school could teach from this book to help improve health outcomes of kids, we hope that you will advocate for a broader use of the 28 lessons so that children will be exposed to many school, home, and community experiences over a three-year time period.

Time and Sequence Guidelines
The sequence of our curriculum includes two units for first graders (10 weeks); three units for second graders (14 weeks), and three units for third graders (18 weeks). These time lines can be flexible as determined by your local curriculum and schedule. Each unit has multiple activities from which to teach the content. However, we hope that the critical concepts and health-related skills remain the focal points of each unit. We also hope that your students have the opportunity to read all 227 picture books over the three-year sequencing. These books have been selected for their health-related storylines, and they may also help to increase health literacy, science literacy, and literacy in general.

Health Literacy
The National Health Education Standards (Joint Committee, 1995, p 6) define health literacy as "the capacity of individuals to obtain, interpret and understand basic health information and services in ways which enhance health". The seven standards serve as a framework for curriculum outcomes which enable students to develop as critical thinkers and problem solvers; responsible, productive citizens; self-directed learners; and effective communicators. The extent to which teachers work to implement *Literature Links for Nutrition and Health* across grades in a collaborative way with other teacher colleagues, parents, food service professionals, librarians, and community organizations, the more that health literacy may be realized. If teachers fail to discuss and demonstrate the multiple connections to health and literacy, then students may not understand how to make health-related decisions between school, home, and community contexts.

Scientific Literacy

The National Science Education Standards promotes scientific literacy, which "enables people to use scientific principles and processes in making personal decisions and to participate in discussions of scientific issues that affect society" (National Research Council, 1996, p. ix). This book can help to advance the science standard which focuses on personal health, especially how it promotes inquiry-based models in which "a person can ask, find, or determine answers to questions derived from curiosity about everyday experiences" (National Research Council, 1996, p 22).

Multiple Intelligence Theory as the Instructional Framework

As discussed above, this book uses national standards documents as a curriculum framework for what students will know and be able to do. Now we need to explain our instruction and assessment model. We believe that health education resources should show connections between curriculum, instruction, and assessment components. Multiple intelligences theory (Gardner, 1983) is an excellent choice for linking instruction and assessment components throughout our four literature-based units. Multiple intelligences theory recognizes that individuals have multiple ways of knowing through which they come to understand the world. As an instructional framework, multiple intelligences offer teachers and students many options for teaching and learning. The seven multiple intelligences are labeled in parentheses throughout each unit to remind you that the ways of knowing and the ways of teaching are related.

The two personal intelligences known as intrapersonal/introspective (I/I) and interpersonal/social (I/S) form the basis for the solo work, small group work, and whole class work in our 28 lessons. The other five intelligences are verbal/linguistic (V/L); logical/mathematical (L/M); visual/spatial (V/S); bodily/kinesthetic (B/K); and musical/rhythmical (M/R). We integrate these five intelligences across the solo work, small group work, and whole class work also. We incorporate all seven intelligences in Across the Curriculum. However, if you are new to multiple intelligences theory, do not confuse multiple ways of knowing with multiple disciplines (Gardner, 1995). For example, a social studies activity may involve the B/K intelligence even though B/K seems to be a prevalent way of knowing in physical education. Like all disciplines, health education can be taught through *all* seven intelligences. You wouldn't use all seven intelligences every day in a health education lesson, but over the course of several days, you should address the multiple ways of knowing and teaching. Health education units which promote multiple intelligences are better able to meet learning outcomes of students with diverse needs, interests, and abilities.

Assessments are Coordinated by the Teacher

Assessment options are provided in our introductory unit 1 so that teachers and faculty will be reminded that decisions about curriculum, instruction, and assessment need to be closely coordinated and informed by each other. The tri-assessment model by Fogarty & Stoehr (1995) offers the option of using traditional, portfolio, and performance assessments for evaluating the health-related topics, concepts, and skills your students will learn during each unit. Ongoing assessments during a unit help to answer questions like "Did this lesson (unit) make a difference in the knowledge, attitudes, and/or behaviors of my students?" and "Did this unit help my students to practice and demonstrate health-related skills of decision making, communication, and goal setting related to health, nutrition, and eating behavior?" Rather than offering a traditional assessment at the end of the unit, we urge you to collect multiple indicators of learning throughout the unit.

Performance indicators are especially germane to health education. For example, we all *know* that we should eat fruits and vegetables each day, but how many of us *do* it? How many students can *demonstrate* that they can select two fruits and three vegetables from a produce stand? Shouldn't that "performance" be equal to a written test at the end of the unit?

Unit Overview
Literature Links for Nutrition and Health is a sequential curriculum for enhancing nutrition knowledge and eating behaviors of children in grades one through three. The scope and sequence chart in Unit 1 specifies the amount of time that is needed to teach the 12 focused themes in the curriculum. For ease in implementation, the time specified for teaching the curriculum is organized by both weeks and months. Try to view the units as sequential building blocks to higher-level concepts and applications. For example, Unit 2 is a foundation to Units 3, 4, and 5. Unit 3 is a foundation to Units 4 and 5, and so forth. Within each unit, you can begin with any focused theme so it fits with your local curriculum and instructional needs. However, we hope that you will teach all of the themes within a unit so that students gain the proper scope and sequence over the course of three years. Nutrition concepts are intended to move from simple to complex and from concrete to abstract during the three years that your students are exposed to the curriculum.

We have four literature-based units which present 28 feature books across 12 focused themes. Each unit begins with suggested lessons for a featured picture book which helps to correlate the focused themes in the unit. For example, unit 5, World of People, has two focused themes called Multigenerational Gatherings and Multicultural Connections, which are introduced through one feature book called *Dumpling Soup* (Rattigan, 1993). After the lesson for *Dumpling Soup*, the unit introduces each of the focused themes with additional picture books and accompanying lessons. Additional literature is organized in each unit in two sections entitled: For the Pleasure of Reading and Other Books to Read. These primary and secondary resources, respectively, give students more books to read in the classroom or at home for reinforcing health-related concepts and skills.

Unit 1 introduces the curriculum, instruction, and assessment frameworks for the book. Unit 2 is called Building the Food Pyramid. This unit has six focused themes which are associated with the five food groups and the non-food group called Fats, Oils, & Sweets of the Food Guide Pyramid. Lessons for each of the six focused themes help to develop concepts from grade to grade. For example, a <u>variety</u> of foods is presented as the concept for grade 1; <u>moderation</u> of food choices is presented as the concept for grade 2, and <u>serving size</u> is presented as the concept for grade 3. Unit 3 is called Let's Make A Meal. There are three focused themes for this unit which investigates the when and where aspects of eating behavior. Grade 1 studies the focused theme of Breakfast, Lunch, and Dinner. Grade 2 explores different places to buy, make, or obtain food in Markets, Bakeries, and Vendors. And Grade 3 investigates the similarities and differences between Diners, Restaurants, and Soup Kitchens. Unit 4 is called Cycle of Life. Second-grade students learn that plant foods and animal foods come from Down on the Farm, a focused theme which also addresses family life of rural America. Unit 5 is called A World of People. Third graders will study two focused themes: Multigenerational Gatherings and Multicultural Connections. Lessons in this unit emphasize the social and cultural aspects of eating, especially the special celebrations that friends and families share during holidays and events.

There are detailed, ready-to-use lessons for each of the 28 feature books in *Literature Links for Nutrition and Health*. Lesson plans for Units 3, 4, and 5 are organized in the following sequence:

Cover Page
⇒ The Name, Author, and Publisher of the Feature Book
⇒ How the lesson addresses the Dietary Guidelines for Americans
⇒ How the lesson highlights the food groups from the Food Guide Pyramid

Lesson Plans
⇒ Pre-Reading Activities for the Feature Book
⇒ Post-Reading Activities for the Feature Book based on Bloom's Taxonomy
⇒ Solo Work for the Feature Book
⇒ Small Group Work for the Feature Book
⇒ Whole Class Work for the Feature Book

Across the Curriculum
Includes multidisciplinary connections to Social Studies, Mathematics, Science, Language Arts, Physical Education, Art, and Music. Suggested activities for each subject area are labeled for its' contribution to multiple intelligences as a way of knowing and a way of teaching.

Other Books to Read for the Focused Theme
Includes books that could be used with the lesson plans in the unit because they present similar topics, concepts, or skills in their storylines. The booklist can be used to bring other books into your classroom library, so students can read more broadly about the focused theme.

Letter to Parents and Caregivers
Provides a sample letter for involving parents and caregivers in the lessons of each unit. Each letter briefly overviews the unit and gives parents and caregivers the option of providing supplies and materials for the lessons.

Letter to Food Service Professionals
Provides a sample letter for involving food service professionals from your school in the lessons of each unit. Each letter briefly overviews the unit and gives food service professionals the option of providing supplies, equipment, and materials for the lessons. Sometimes the letters will request the food service professional to speak to the class or assist during a culminating event in the unit.

For the Pleasure of Reading
Includes books that are secondary reading choices for a focused theme. The books are actually primary choices in another unit, but are included again at the end of some units so that students can read books which have multiple connections to food and nutrition concepts. This book list can be shared with parents and caregivers for use as educational enrichments with their children.

Acknowledgements

Collaboration is the true cornerstone of a successful project. Though one or two people carried the day-to-day demands of designing this book and creating its contents, others offered invaluable assistance. A selected cadre of former students who learned about health education and nutrition education in our classes were assistants in this project in both conceptual and practical ways. The involvement of these preservice teachers gave them experiential learning in grant work, library skills, and computer database management. In turn, we engaged in discussions with them about their professional coursework, field work in schools, and student teaching placements in suburban, urban, and rural settings. We greatly appreciate Jocelyn Weeda, Sarah Inglis, Debra Butanowicz Majeski, Suzanne Moore, Tonia Ricketts Kennedy, and Allison Bucci Kelly. We thank Amy Mallory, Elisa Dugan, Joanne Hannaway, Kelley Chupka Flaugher, Krista Saylor, and Melissa McCoy. And we also acknowledge the dedication of four graduate students: Kim Shafer, Jennifer Brown, Sally Bayes-Foxx, and especially, Kerry Gray, whose standards of quality were invaluable to our project.

We thank Meg Wagner, MS, RD, LD, for funding our initial project ideas through the Nutrition Education and Training (NET) Program, Ohio Department of Education, Columbus, OH. Thank you to Vicki Striggow Salisbury, MS, RD, and Vickie L. Douglas, PhD, CHES, who shared helpful and timely nutrition resources without being asked. We also appreciate the professional ideas of Garry R. Bowyer, PhD, our colleague in the Department of Physical Education, Health, and Sport Studies. We are especially indebted to Bill Ubbes for his technical support in managing the acquisition of computer equipment, installation of software and hardware, daily back-ups, and trouble-shooting computer problems. The project was enhanced by his wisdom, editorial finesse, trademark good humor, and perspectives on the important things in life.

It is important to reflect on why health education, nutrition education, and elementary education have come together at this juncture in my life. My earliest professional mentor, Nancy Ray Striggow (Mom), had a wonderful career in physical education and home economics in public schools. Mom moved easily across disciplines and saw connections between the classroom, gymnasium, school, and home -- a philosophy that I promote in higher education. My mom raised seven children during her career. Though some may regard it as a challenge for me to have undertaken this project while my own children were so young, Allegra and Joshua have been a constant source of inspiration. This book is much more relevant because of my joyful children. My children love books and are part of a greater family of book lovers. My mother-in-law, Dorothy Schlobohm Ubbes, opened many childrens' eyes to the world of books as a first grade teacher. She continues to do so during her retirement years by tutoring children who are learning to read. This book has exemplified the quote "Remember that a relationship is a pooling of resources. That means that with each relationship you are not only giving, you are becoming more" (Buscaglia,1984).

Valerie A. Ubbes, PhD, CHES

I want to thank Valerie, my colleague and friend, and acknowledge the inspiration that comes from having her children in our midst when working. I find that children, like Allegra and Joshua, can help you strive to endure and work harder, so that they can have a better world. A world where all people, young and old, can have access to good nutrition and health.

Diana M. Spillman, PhD, RD, LD

Unit 1
Introduction & Background

Literature Links for Nutrition and Health provides you with a nutrition education curriculum for enhancing health knowledge and eating behaviors of your students. Using this nutrition curricula within a coordinated school health program (Marx & Wooley, 1998) will help to ensure that students receive a strong consistent message about healthful eating behaviors from ages five to eight. Specifically, classroom teachers teaching from this curriculum can team with food service professionals, parents, caregivers, community health organizations, certified health education specialists, physical education specialists, registered dietitians, media specialists, and other classroom teachers to effectively implement the sequential lessons from grades one through three. Preservice teachers and dietitians from local colleges and universities can also be excellent resources for helping you to implement the lessons to children in your classroom. Through service learning opportunities, there can be simultaneous renewal between schools and universities in how we come to understand the relationship between curriculum, instruction, and assessment in health education.

This unit will provide you with an introduction to this book and give you background information on curriculum, instruction, and assessment frameworks. We offer you curriculum frameworks, including the National Health Education Standards and several nutrition guidelines which serve as organizers to each unit. We also provide instruction and assessment frameworks through the multiple intelligences and a tri-assessment model, respectively. These frameworks and guidelines provide structure to each unit. However, the accompanying lessons are designed to be flexible and adaptive to local needs and interests. The next section will preview the content of each unit.

Unit Overview

Literature-based lessons in Units 2, 3, 4, and 5 are designed around twelve focused themes. Unit 2, Building the Food Pyramid, explores the major food groups through six focused themes. The remaining six focused themes of Units 3, 4, and 5 are described on the next page.

What is a focused theme? A focused theme introduces one to three featured books as lesson starters in a unit. A featured book is reviewed first for its alignment to the U.S. Dietary Guidelines and Food Guide Pyramid. These guidelines are explained over the next few pages. Then teaching ideas are provided to introduce each book, including follow-up questions about the book. These hierarchical questions, aimed at critical thinking about the storyline, are organized by Bloom's Taxonomy. These question probes can be used throughout the unit each time a picture book is read. Try to read a featured book often during a unit, because children enjoy hearing the same book again and again. Have different people read the book, including teachers, students, and classroom guests. Before teaching from a unit, ask your media specialist and public librarians to locate the other books suggested in each unit. Each focused theme has a booklist called "Other Books to Read for the Focused Theme", and then at the end of each unit, another booklist called "For the Pleasure of Reading" helps to extend literature from school to home. Broadening the use of literature beyond the featured book of a focused theme will really help the classroom, cafeteria, and community lessons come alive when you explore the individual, small group, and whole class projects, including the multidisciplinary connections across the curriculum.

The focused themes for Units 3, 4, and 5 are described below:

Overview of Breakfast, Lunch, and Dinner:

This focused theme in Unit 3 emphasizes our eating behavior during the three major meals of our day, including snacks. Eating behavior is designated by *what* we eat, *when* we eat, *where* we eat, and *with whom* we eat. This section will highlight when we eat. For example, most people eat a morning meal, an afternoon meal, and an evening meal. Some people also eat one or two nutritious snacks during their active day. The feature books in this section also address what kinds of foods and with whom we eat our meals.

Overview of Markets, Bakeries, and Vendors:

This focused theme in Unit 3 highlights three different places where we buy food to eat. Have you ever been to a large market or a mega grocery store? What do you like best about stopping at the bakery for your favorite bread or rolls? Have you ever bought any food on a street corner or roadside stand? The feature books in this section show what kinds of foods we buy when shopping, and the kinds of foods we make after getting home and unloading the grocery bags.

Overview of Diners, Restaurants, and Soup Kitchens:

This focused theme in Unit 3 emphasizes eating behavior in three different public places where food is eaten. Eating behavior is designated by *what* we eat, *when* we eat, *where* we eat, and *with whom* we eat. What food do you eat at your favorite restaurant? Do you like to go with anyone in particular? Do you tend to eat more food or less food when you go out to eat? This section will highlight where we eat. The feature books in this section also address what kinds of foods and with whom we eat our meals.

Overview of Down on the Farm:

This focused theme in Unit 4 looks at where plant foods are grown and harvested and where animal products are produced and marketed. This section also highlights the cycle of life on a farm for plants and animals. Some historical and cultural backgrounds of food are investigated. Since farm life requires hard work, the social and economic aspects of living and working on a farm are explored through several of the featured books.

Overview of Multigenerational Gatherings

This focused theme in Unit 5 highlights the social gatherings we share with people from our families and friends who are from an older generation. We gain a healthy perspective on aging when we share thoughts, feelings, past memories, and current events with people of all ages. Several featured books in this unit show what it's like to grow up with the love and support of people from many generations while sharing everyday activities like meal preparation and eating.

Overview of Multicultural Connections

This focused theme in Unit 5 explores concepts of diversity and culture in the context of food and nutrition. Some similarities and differences surface when we compare how we eat, when we eat, and with whom we eat during celebrations, holidays, and everyday meals. Several featured books show what it's like to prepare and enjoy food with our family and friends of different backgrounds and heritages.

Implementation Schedule for Units 2, 3, 4, & 5

This chart provides a list of all twelve focused themes by unit and by grade level. This implementation schedule is organized by weeks and months, so that you can plan how much time is needed to teach a focused theme and unit.

Name of Focused Theme by Unit	Grade Level	Weeks Needed for Teaching Focused Theme	Months Needed for Teaching Unit in Grade 1	Months Needed for Teaching Unit in Grade 2	Months Needed for Teaching Unit in Grade 3
Unit 2			1.5 months for Grade 1	1.5 months for Grade 2	1.5 months for Grade 3
Bread, Cereal, Rice, & Pasta	Grades 1, 2, & 3	1 week			
Fruit Group	Grades 1, 2, & 3	1 week			
Vegetable Group	Grades 1, 2, & 3	1 week			
Milk, Yogurt, & Cheese Group	Grades 1, 2, & 3	1 week			
Meat, Poultry, Fish, Dry Beans, Eggs, & Nuts	Grades 1, 2, & 3	1 week			
Fats, Oils, & Sweets Group	Grades 1, 2, & 3	1 week			
Unit 3			1 month for Grade 1	1 month for Grade 2	1 month for Grade 3
Breakfast, Lunch, & Dinner	Grade 1	4 weeks			
Markets, Bakeries & Vendors	Grade 2	4 weeks			
Diners, Restaurants & Soup Kitchens	Grade 3	4 weeks			
Unit 4				1 month for Grade 2	
Down on the Farm	Grade 2	4 weeks			
Unit 5					2 months for Grade 3
Multigenerational Gatherings	Grade 3	4 weeks			
Multicultural Connections	Grade 3	4 weeks			

The next page shows how each unit is aligned to the National Health Education Standards.

Curriculum Framework: National Health Education Standards

National Health Education Standards for Grades K-12	Met by Unit 2 Instructional Activities (Grades 1-3)	Met by Unit 3 Instructional Activities (Grades 1-3)	Met by Unit 4 Instructional Activities (Grade 2)	Met by Unit 5 Instructional Activities (Grade 3)
Students will comprehend concepts related to health promotion and disease prevention.	X	X	X	X
Students will demonstrate the ability to access valid health information and health promotion products and services.	X	X		
Students will demonstrate the ability to practice health-enhancing behaviors and reduce health risks.	X	X	X	
Students will analyze the influence of culture, media, technology, and other factors on health.		X	X	X
Students will demonstrate the ability to use interpersonal communication skills to enhance health.		X	X	X
Students will demonstrate the ability the use goal setting and decision-making skills to enhance health.	X	X	X	X
Students will demonstrate the ability to advocate for personal, family, and community health.	X	X	X	X

Dietary Guidelines for Americans

The *Dietary Guidelines for Americans (1995)*, issued every five years by the U.S. Department of Agriculture and the U.S. Department of Health and Human Services, is a guide that provides practical advise for healthy Americans age 2 years and over about food choices that promote health and prevent disease. The objective of the *Dietary Guidelines for Americans* is to promote healthful dietary practices and to reduce the risk of chronic and degenerative diseases in the population. The guidelines are listed below:

The ***Dietary Guidelines for Americans include:***

1. **Eat a variety of foods.** Obtain the many nutrients your body needs by choosing a variety of foods you enjoy from each of the Five Food Groups.

2. **Balance the food you eat with physical activity; maintain or improve your weight.** Try to maintain body weight by balancing what you eat with physical activity. More physical activity is better than less, and any is better than none. Take steps to keep your weight within a healthy range.

3. **Choose a diet with plenty of grain products, vegetables, and fruits.** These foods are the foundation of a healthful diet; they provide vitamins, minerals, complex carbohydrates (starch and dietary fiber), and other substances that are important for good health.

4. **Choose a diet low in fat, saturated fat, and cholesterol.** For adults, no more than 30% of total calories should come from fat and less than 10% of total calories from saturated fat. For infants and toddlers below the age of 2, no restrictions apply. The guideline does recommend that children, by about age 5, gradually adopt a diet that contains no more than 30% of total calories from fat.

5. **Choose a diet moderate in sugars**. This guideline has not changed since the 1990 edition. Moderation is still the key!

6. **Choose a diet moderate in salt and sodium.** Processed, prepared, and preserved foods are the source of most dietary sodium, not salt from the salt shaker.

7. **If you drink alcoholic beverages, do so in moderation.** Alcohol supplies calories but few, if any, nutrients. Moderation is no more than 1 drink per day for women, and no more than 2 drinks per day for men. This guideline does not pertain to children and youth who are minors.

Variety, balance, and moderation continue to be the foundation of a healthful diet.

The *Dietary Guidelines for Americans* can be accessed electronically from the World Wide Web. Visit the following sites:
http://www.nalusda.gov/fnic./dga/dguide95.html
http://www.nalusda.gov/fnic./dga/dga95.html
http://www.usda.gov:80/cnpp/dietary_guidelines.htm

Food Guide Pyramid

Developed by the U.S. Department of Agriculture and supported by the U.S. Department of Health and Human Services, the *Food Guide Pyramid* takes the *Dietary Guidelines for Americans* one step further. The pyramid model provides a framework for eating a variety of foods in order to ensure an adequate intake of nutrients, while cutting down on fat, sugar, and sodium, and maintaining a healthy weight. The Pyramid classifies food into five major food groups. Each of these food groups provides some, but not all, of the nutrients you need. Foods in one group can't replace those in another. No one food group is more important than another — for good health, you need them all. The sixth category, though not considered a Food Group, consists of Fats, Oils, & Sweets. Foods that contain these items should be used sparingly in your diet. A copy of the Food Guide Pyramid is provided below. Food Guide Pyramid information can also be accessed at http://warp.nal.usda.gov:80/fnic/Fpyr/pyramid.html and http://www.usda.gov/cnpp/KidsPyra/index.htm

The five major food groups of the Food Guide Pyramid are:
Bread, Cereal, Rice, & Pasta Group
Fruit Group
Vegetable Group
Milk, Yogurt, & Cheese Group
Meat, Poultry, Fish, Dry Beans, Eggs, & Nuts Group

The sixth category of the Pyramid is:
Fats, Oils, & Sweet

Food Guide Pyramid
A Guide to Daily Food Choices

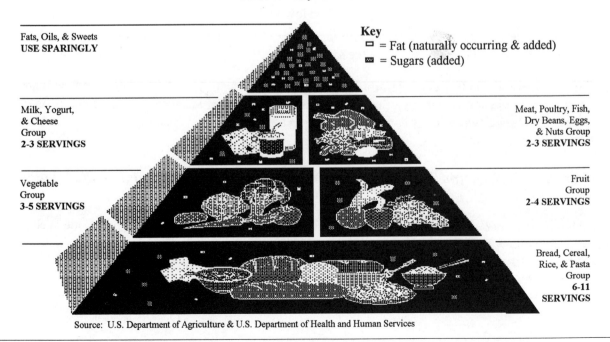

Source: U.S. Department of Agriculture & U.S. Department of Health and Human Services

Selected School-Based Strategies to Promote Healthy Eating

Selected School-Based Strategies to Promote Healthy Eating (U.S. Centers for Disease Control and Prevention, 1996) are guidelines aimed at promoting lifelong healthy eating patterns among school-age children and youth. The strategies suggest ways to make the food environment in schools more health-enhancing and to support healthy eating among children. The following guidelines may be helpful to your school:

Strategies to make the food environment in schools more health-enhancing

- Make healthy foods (e.g., fruits, vegetables, and whole grains) widely available at school, and discourage the availability of foods high in fat, sodium, and added sugars.

- Involve parents in nutrition education through homework.

- Provide role models (e.g., teachers, parents, other adults, older children, and celebrities or fictional characters) for healthy eating.

- Provide cues, through posters and marketing-style incentives, that encourage students to make healthy choices about eating and physical activity.

- Use incentives, such as verbal praise or token gifts, to reinforce healthy eating and physical activity. Do not use food for reward or punishment of any behavior.

Strategies to support healthy eating among children

- Make basic connections between food and health, e.g.,"You need food to feel good and to grow".

- Teach the importance of balancing food intake and physical activity.

- Identify healthy snacks, e.g., fruits, vegetables, and low-fat milk.

- Increase students' confidence in their ability to make healthy eating choices by gradually building up their food selection and preparation skills and giving them practice.

- Provide many healthy foods for students to taste in an enjoyable social context.

- Let students prepare simple snacks.

- Have students try unfamiliar and culturally diverse foods that are low in fat, sodium, and added sugars.

You may also view a companion document, *Guidelines for School Health Programs to Promote Lifelong Healthy Eating,* electronically at http://www.cdc.gov/nccdphp/dash/guide.htm

Instruction and Assessment Frameworks for Each Unit

This section provides you with blackline templates for Units 2, 3, 4, and 5. These templates may be photocopied for each unit to help you with the following:

⇒ Overview of the Multiple Intelligences

The multiple intelligences describe the multiple ways of knowing about the world. The template on the next page provides guiding questions to help you make choices about instructional methodology (pedagogy) in each unit. As described in the preface, multiple intelligences are listed in parentheses behind each of the teaching ideas within a lesson. These help you to know that the lesson has the potential to meet the diverse learning needs of your students;

⇒ Assessment Web of Multiple Intelligences for the Unit

This web can be used as a template to showcase the parts of lessons you selected to teach from each unit. During the unit study, use the assessment web to write the different lesson ideas that you used for each of the intelligences. You can then use your selections to determine assessments before, during, and after the unit is implemented to answer the questions: "What will students know and be able to do as a result of this unit?" The next model will show how your instruction and assessment decisions can be coordinated;

⇒ Tri-Assessment Model: Traditional, Portfolio, and Performance Assessments

This framework provides a way of thinking about the different ways of knowing (intelligences) and the different ways of assessing teaching and learning. The bottom of this page asks "how will you assess your students during each unit? Four questions at the bottom of the template will help you to organize your assessment plan for the unit;

⇒ Assessment Plan for Each Unit

This sample assessment plan is a graphic organizer for determining which assessment options will work best for the concepts and skills in a unit. The sample template draws upon the Unit 2 concepts of variety, moderation, and serving size. This form can be repeated for other units too; and

⇒ Final Assessment of the Overall Featured Book in Each Unit

This sample assessment plan helps to review the overall featured book of each unit. We provide an example for Unit 2 for you to consider. Select one type of assessment from the three options to assess your students' understanding of the book. We hope that you will especially consider performance assessments, because they help to assess content and process simultaneously.

Overview of the Multiple Intelligences

As a teacher, you know that students have unique ways of learning and multiple ways of knowing. Multiple intelligence theory can be used as a way of knowing, a way of teaching, and a way of assessing learning. You won't always find ways to include every intelligence in a particular lesson. But maybe the questions (Armstrong, 1987) and the model (Gardner, 1983) below will help you plan for one or two intelligences that you may not have considered!

Intrapersonal/Introspective: How can I evoke personal feelings, memories, and give students choices? How does self reflection play a role?

Verbal/Linguistic: How can I use the spoken and written word?

Musical/Rhythmical: How can I bring in music and environmental sounds, and set key content to a rhythm or melody?

Logical/Mathematical: How can I use numbers, calculations, classifications, logic, and critical thinking for exploration of patterns, categories, and relationships?

Bodily/Kinesthetic: How can I help students learn by moving and acting things out? How can I involve the whole body and hands-on experiences?

Interpersonal/Social: How can I engage students in peer or cross-age sharing, cooperative learning, and large-group simulations?

Visual/Spatial: How can I use visual aids, visualizations, color, art, metaphors, and graphic organizers?

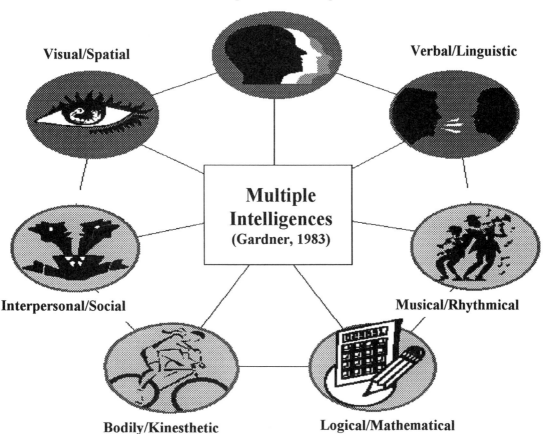

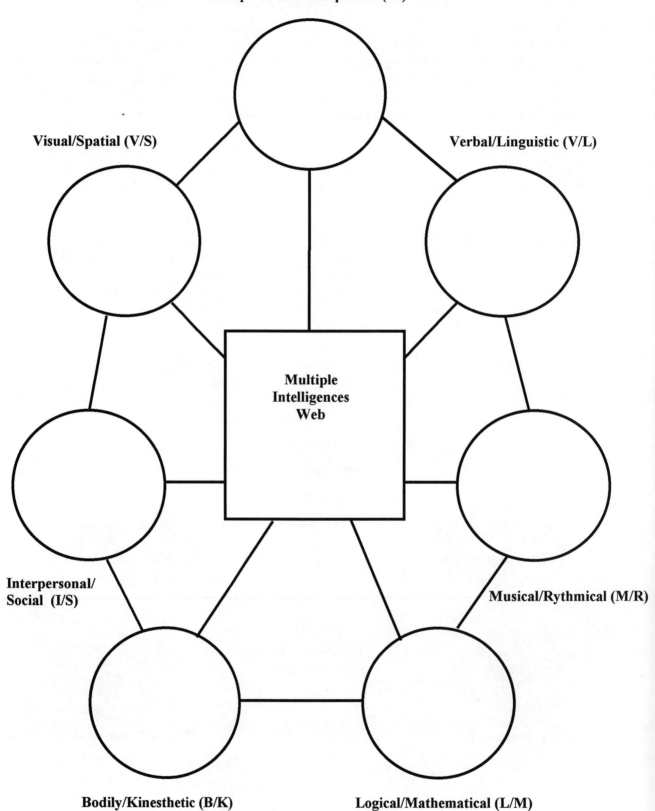

Tri-Assessment Model (Fogarty & Stoehr, 1995)

Reprinted by permission of SkyLight Training and Publishing, Inc. Arlington Heights, IL.

Multiple Intelligences	Types of Assessment	Focus of Assessment	Assessment Methods
Verbal/Linguistic Mathematical/Logical Visual/Spatial	Traditional Assessment	Grades and Rankings	Classwork Homework Criterion Referenced Norm Referenced
Verbal/Linguistic Mathematical/Logical Visual/Spatial Intrapersonal/Introspective Interpersonal/Social	Portfolio Assessment	Growth and Development	Collection Selection Reflection Inspection
Verbal/Linguistic Mathematical/Logical Visual/Spatial Interpersonal/Social Bodily/Kinesthetic Musical/Rhythmic	Performance Assessment	Relevance and Transfer	Scoring Rubrics Standards Criteria Indicators

How Will You Assess Your Students During Each Unit?

Directions: The first two columns in the chart above describe whether an intelligence can be evaluated by traditional, portfolio, or performance assessment. Select **one** activity from your Multiple Intelligences Web for the unit and write it below. Next list the type of intelligence the activity develops and which type of assessment you plan to do for the selected activity. Write a short description of your planning steps needed to evaluate your students.

Selected Activity from this Unit:_____

Multiple Intelligence that the Activity Develops:_____

Will you use Traditional, Portfolio, or Performance Assessment? _____

Describe Your Assessment: _____

Assessment Plan For Each Unit

What are the main concepts from Unit 2 that you will use to evaluate your students at a grade level?	What **Traditional** Assessments will you use to assess your students? What concept should they know? What skill should they be able to do?	What **Portfolio** Assessments will you use to assess your students? What concept should they know? What skill should they be able to do?	What **Performance** Assessments will you use to assess your students? What concept should they know? What skill should they be able to do?
Grade 1 Concept: **Variety of Food**			
Grade 2 Concept: **Moderation**			
Grade 3 Concept: **Serving Size**			

Final Assessment of Overall Featured Book

Directions: As a class or individually, reread *The Edible Pyramid* which is the Feature Book for this unit. In the section below, choose **one** type of assessment from which to test your students' understanding of the book. For Traditional Assessment, you could develop a paper-and-pencil test to evaluate your students' ability to answer the discussion questions (Bloom's Taxonomy) for this book. For Portfolio Assessment, your students could create a private or class collection of items that are mentioned in the storyline. Or your students could write a narrative that describes how they feel about what they learned or how they have used the information from the book to improve or maintain their health. For Performance Assessment, your students could perform a role play or demonstration that exhibits certain nutrition or health-skills related to the book. Write your plan for one of the items below. If you chose Traditional Assessment for the first graders or Performance Assessment for the second graders in your school, then you might select Portfolio Assessment for the third graders. *The Edible Pyramid* can and should be repeated as the Feature Book for three years in a row, because the major concepts of emphasis change from year to year in the unit. This encourages you to team with other teachers so you select a different type of final assessment for students over their first, second, and third grade years.

Traditional Assessment:

Portfolio Assessment:

Performance Assessment:

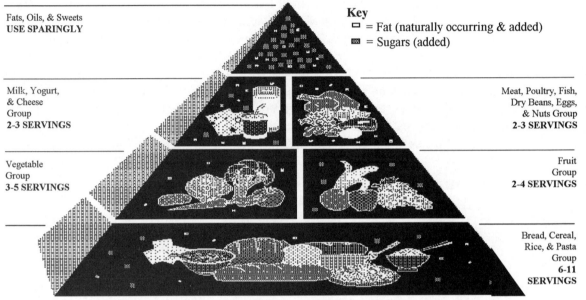

Food Guide Pyramid
A Guide to Daily Food Choices

Fats, Oils, & Sweets
USE SPARINGLY

Key
□ = Fat (naturally occurring & added)
▨ = Sugars (added)

Milk, Yogurt,
& Cheese
Group
2-3 SERVINGS

Meat, Poultry, Fish,
Dry Beans, Eggs,
& Nuts Group
2-3 SERVINGS

Vegetable
Group
3-5 SERVINGS

Fruit
Group
2-4 SERVINGS

Bread, Cereal,
Rice, & Pasta
Group
**6-11
SERVINGS**

Source: U.S. Department of Agriculture & U.S. Department of Health and Human Services

Unit 2:
<u>Building the Food Pyramid</u>

Bread, Cereal, Rice, & Pasta Group
Fruit Group
Vegetable Group
Milk, Yogurt, & Cheese Group
Meat, Poultry, Fish, Beans, Eggs, & Nuts Group
Fats, Oils, & Sweets

Unit 2: Building the Food Pyramid

Instructional activities for Unit 2 have been designed to achieve the *National Health Education Standards* as shown in bold-face type:

$\Rightarrow$ 2. **Students will demonstrate the ability to access valid health information and health-promotion products and services.**
Performance Indicators:
As a result of health instruction in Grades K-4, students will:
1. Identify characteristics of valid health information and health-promoting products and services.

$\Rightarrow$ 3. **Students will demonstrate the ability to practice health-enhancing behaviors and reduce health risks.**
Performance Indicators:
As a result of health instruction in Grades K-4, students will:
1. Identify responsible health behaviors.
2. Identify personal health needs.
4. Demonstrate strategies to improve or maintain personal health.

$\Rightarrow$ 6. **Students will demonstrate the ability to use goal setting and decision-making skills to enhance health.**
Performance Indicators:
As a result of health instruction in Grades K-4, students will:
1. demonstrate the ability to apply a decision-making process to health issues and problems.

$\Rightarrow$ 7. **Students will demonstrate the ability to advocate for personal, family, and community health.**
Performance Indicators:
As a result of health instruction in Grades K-4, students will:
2. express information and opinions about health issues.
4. demonstrate the ability to influence and support others in making positive health choices.

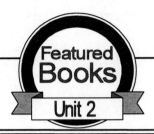

Overall Featured Book for Unit 2

Leedy, L. (1994). The edible pyramid: Good eating every day. New York: Holiday House.
   The Edible Pyramid restaurant opens as the maitre d' explains the food
   pyramid menu to the customers. The maitre d' discusses which foods are
   included in each group. He also discusses how many servings from each
   group should be eaten everyday. Beginning reading level.

Book for Focused Theme: Bread, Cereal, Rice, & Pasta Group

Morris, A. (1989). Bread, bread, bread. New York: Scholastic Inc.
   Bread comes in many sizes and shapes and is eaten by people all over the world. Bread helps
   you grow and makes you strong. Look at all the different cultures that use bread!
   (Non-fiction). Beginning reading level.

Book for Focused Theme: Fruit Group

Lember, B. H. (1994). A book of fruit. New York: Ticknor and Fields Books.
   Pictures show where all different fruits grow. For example, apples in an apple orchard and
   berries in the berry patch. (Non-fiction). Beginning reading level.

Book for Focused Theme: Vegetable Group

de Bourgoing & Jeunesse, G. (1989). Vegetables in the garden. New York: Cartwheel Books.
   This book shows a cross-sectional view of various vegetables. Carrots, radishes, beets,
   potatoes and zucchini are a few of the incredible edibles in this book. (Non-fiction).
   Intermediate reading level.

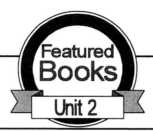

Book for Focused Theme: Milk, Yogurt, & Cheese Group

Aliki. (1992). Milk from cow to carton. New York: HarperCollins Children's Books.
Describes the steps of milking a cow then processing it at a dairy. Children also learn how butter and cheese are made from milk. (Non-fiction). Advanced reading level.

Book for Focused Theme: Meat, Poultry, Fish, Dry Beans, Eggs, & Nuts Group

Cohen, P. &. L. O. (1989). Olson's meat pies. New York: R & S Books.
Olson makes meat pies with the best ingredients. One day Olsen's bookkeeper runs off with all of his money. Olson is forced to put strange ingredients in the pies -- like watches. When the bookkeeper comes back with most of Olson's money, the meat pies are good again. Advanced reading level.

Book for Focused Theme: Fats, Oils, & Sweets Group

Wagner, K. (1990). Chocolate chip cookies. New York: Henry Holt & Co., Inc.
Two little boys show how to make chocolate chip cookies through a set of one word instructions. Beginning reading level.

Unit 2: Building the Food Pyramid
Scope & Sequence of Nutrition Content

Grades 1, 2, & 3

Nutrition Content: Dietary Guidelines	*The Edible Pyramid: Good Eating Every Day*	*Bread, Bread, Bread*	*A Book of Fruit*	*Vegetables in the Garden*	*Milk from Cow to Carton*	*Olson's Meat Pies*	*Chocolate Chip Cookies*
Eat a variety of foods	X	X	X	X			
Balance food with exercise	X						
Choose grains, vegetables, and fruits	X	X	X	X			
Choose low fat and low cholesterol	X				X	X	X
Choose moderate sugars	X						X
Choose moderate salt/sodium							

Nutrition Content: Food Groups	*The Edible Pyramid: Good Eating Every Day*	*Bread, Bread, Bread*	*A Book of Fruit*	*Vegetables in the Garden*	*Milk From Cow to Carton*	*Olson's Meat Pies*	*Chocolate Chip Cookies*
Bread, Cereal, Rice, & Pasta Group	X	X					
Fruit Group	X		X				
Vegetable Group	X			X		X	
Milk, Yogurt, & Cheese Group	X				X		
Meat, Poultry, Fish, Beans, Eggs, & Nuts Group	X					X	
Fats, Oils, & Sweets Group	X						X

The Edible Pyramid
by Loreen Leedy
Holiday House, 1994

This lesson addresses the following Dietary Guidelines for Americans:

⇒ *1. Eat a variety of foods.*
⇒ *2. Balance the food you eat with physical activity; maintain or improve your weight.*
⇒ *3. Choose a diet with plenty of grain products, vegetables, and fruits.*
⇒ *4. Choose a diet low in fat, saturated fat, and cholesterol.*
⇒ *5. Choose a diet moderate in sugars.*
6. Choose a diet moderate in salt and sodium.
7. Choose an alcohol and drug-free lifestyle.

This lesson highlights the following food groups from the Food Guide Pyramid:

⇒ *Bread, Cereal, Rice, & Pasta Group*
⇒ *Fruit Group*
⇒ *Vegetable Group*
⇒ *Milk, Yogurt, & Cheese Group*
⇒ *Meat, Poultry, Fish, Dry Beans, Eggs, & Nuts Group*
⇒ *Fats, Oils, & Sweets*

Food Guide Pyramid
A Guide to Daily Food Choices

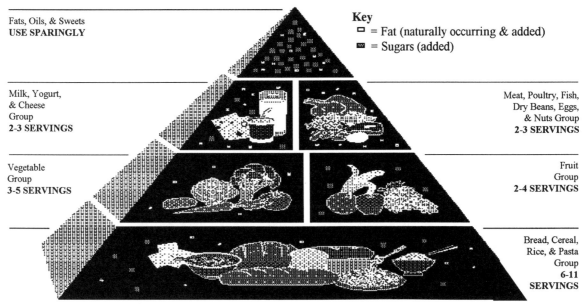

Source: U.S. Department of Agriculture & U.S. Department of Health and Human Services

Lesson Plans for Overall Featured Book

Leedy, L. (1994). The edible pyramid: Good eating every day. New York: Holiday House.
The Edible Pyramid restaurant opens as the maitre d' explains the food
pyramid menu to the customers. The maitre d' discusses which foods are
included in each group. He also discusses how many servings from each
group should be eaten everyday. Beginning reading level.

Pre-Reading Activities for *The Edible Pyramid*

Nutrition is the science of how the body uses food (Evers, 1995). Look up the word "nutrition" in several books, including dictionaries, encyclopedias, and cookbooks. Compare at least 5 different definitions for the word "nutrition". What definition will your class use?

How does a triangle and pyramid compare? Describe some characteristics of each. Why is the Food Guide Pyramid a good visual for guiding our food choices each day?

Post-Reading Activities for *The Edible Pyramid*

Questions to develop thinking skills (Bloom's Taxonomy)

1. Knowledge: Repeat the names of the five food groups in the book.

2. Comprehension: Restate how sizes are determined.

3. Application: Report all of the foods you have eaten so far today. Have you had at least one serving from each food group discussed in the book?

4. Analysis: Compare the food groups on the food pyramid. Which groups contain more servings? What conclusions can you draw about these differences?

5. Synthesis: Plan a nutritionally balanced meal for yourself at this restaurant. What would you eat for breakfast? Lunch? Dinner? A snack?

6. Evaluation: Choose three animal characters in the book. Consider the differences and similarities between food eaten by people and food eaten by animals.

Solo Work for *The Edible Pyramid*

Give five 4" x 6" index cards to each student. Have students write the name of one of the food groups on an index card. Be sure to spell all the words correctly and to write the complete name of the food group. Repeat for the other four food groups. For first graders, make a template of one set of food group cards on several pieces of paper, then photocopy them for each member of your class. Help students to cut their food group cards with scissors and read each card outloud. Set the cards aside until the Whole Class Work activity below.

Small Group Work for *The Edible Pyramid*

Write to several organizations to obtain a poster, a refrigerator magnet, or three-dimensional model of the Food Guide Pyramid for use in class during this unit. Each small group of students can draft a letter to a different organization requesting different pyramid materials. Addresses and phone numbers of these organizations are located in the back of this book. One student can address the envelope, one student can write the letter with everyone's input, and one student can proof the letter for accuracy. All students should sign the letter. For first graders, the class can draft a letter together while the teacher writes on the board or easel paper. If your class has a telephone in the room and a speaker phone, the teacher or a student volunteer can place a toll-free call to one or more of the organizations to request their materials. Phone requests are usually filled faster than mail requests.

While waiting for the material to arrive, begin to work through the major concepts of this unit by:
1) Agreeing upon definitions for the words: *variety* (first graders), *moderation* (second graders), and *serving size* (third graders). Use different dictionaries to help you. Each small group should write their definitions on a 4" x 6" index card and submit them to their teacher. All the cards can then be compared and discussed so the class will understand the term before completing the whole class work below.

Whole Class Work for *The Edible Pyramid*

Students are now prepared to talk about the different levels of the food pyramid. An initial orientation to the food groups might be simplified into three levels from bottom to top as follows:
Level I:
The **Bread, Cereal, Rice, and Pasta Group** can be called the Grain Group which consists of *energy foods*.
Level II:
The **Vegetable Group** can be called the Vegetable Group which consists of *maintenance foods*.
The **Fruit Group** can be called the Fruit Group which consists of *maintenance foods*.
Level III:
The **Milk, Yogurt & Cheese Group** can be called the Dairy Group which consists of *body-building foods*.
The **Meat, Poultry, Fish, Dry Beans, Eggs, and Nuts Group** can be called the Protein Group which consists of *body-building foods*.
Level IV:
The **Fats, Oils, & Sweets Group** can be called the Other Group which consists of *caution foods*.
This group is usually not referred to as one of the five food groups; it is an extra category.

Help students to write the italicized words listed above on the back of their individual Food Group cards. Use these flashcards to learn the name and spelling of each food group, to categorize and label foods in class, and sort students into groups for activities. These strategies will be explained throughout this unit.

Across the Curriculum

Across the Curriculum for *The Edible Pyramid*

Social Studies

Food Pyramids exist for many different cultures. Preview the different multicultural food guide pyramids shown throughout Unit 5. There's quite a variety of foods from which to choose. Also go to the World Wide Web to look at the variety of food guide pyramids available @ http://www.warp.nal.usda.gov:80/fnic/etext/000023.html

Mathematics

Have you ever noticed that the food pyramid encourages you to drink milk, fruit juice, and vegetable juice, but it doesn't mention anything about water? Water is the most essential nutrient in our diet and is a compound made up of two chemicals — oxygen and hydrogen. Our bodies need water in order to metabolize food, breath, and rid the body of waste products. A rule of thumb is to drink one cup (8 ounces) of water eight times each day. First graders can practice filling 8 cups of water into a pitcher to see how many ounces that makes. Second graders can experiment with the concept of volume by looking at how one cup of water (8 ounces) "looks" in a tall glass versus a short glass. Third graders can try to calculate how many gulps of water at the drinking faucet makes one cup of water (8 ounces).

Science

What makes a fruit a fruit? Or what makes a vegetable a vegetable? How do you know if a tomato is a fruit or a vegetable? What are the parts of a plant that we eat? There are six parts to edible plants: seeds, roots, stems, leaves, flowers, and fruits. Coordinate a display in the cafeteria that shows food examples for each category. First graders can show food examples of seeds and roots; second graders can show food examples of stems and leaves; and third graders can show food examples of flowers and fruits. Invite your local supermarket to donate the food for your display then take some photos to post in the store afterwards to increase awareness about the edible parts of plants. Don't forget to invite your principal and superintendent to eat lunch with your class on the day that you display your Plant Food. Yum! Yum!

Language Arts

There are many nutrition-related celebrations each month across the country. For example, there's the American Heart Month in February; National Nutrition Month and National School Breakfast Week in March; Dairy Month in June; National Cholesterol Education Month in September; and National School Lunch Week and World Food Day in October. Ask your food service professionals which celebrations they plan to promote in your school, then volunteer your class to write or call for promotional information to distribute to other teachers and students in your building. Knowing who to ask and where to find addresses and phone numbers is half the fun. You can also try accessing a list from http://nhic-nt.health.org/pubs/99hfinders/index.html.

Across the Curriculum for *The Edible Pyramid, continued*

Physical Education

Your body uses energy from food when you exercise. Can you think of any movements that we can do that are fast and intense? Slow and easy? Movements that are fast and intense tend to use carbohydrate-rich foods to help your muscles contract. Carbohydrate-rich foods come from three* of the five food groups: grains group, vegetable group, and fruit group. Think of a cheer with lots of fast and intense movements to celebrate the Grains Group (first graders), Vegetable Group (second graders), and Fruit Group (third graders). Hold a special pep assembly at the end of your school day in the cafeteria to demonstrate your cheers. With a little creativity you can get everyone active in the cheer. Be safety conscious as you actively participate. Go-go-go-go grains!

*Some carbohydrates are also present in the Milk, Yogurt, & Cheese Group. However, the majority of energy in this food group comes from proteins and fats.

Art

To raise awareness about the benefits of the Food Guide Pyramid, make place mats to use in the cafeteria during your School Breakfast and School Lunch programs. Laminate them so they last longer than one meal. First graders might choose one food group to draw and label. Divide your total class by five groups to get the number of students creating placemats for one food group. Second graders can draw a lunch or dinner plate graphic in the middle of their personal placemats in order to show healthful meal choices. Cut and paste food pictures from magazines to create two-dimensional placemats. Foods should be selected and assembled on the basis of variety and moderation. Third graders can make placemats that show different serving sizes. Divide your total class by five groups to get the number of students creating placemats for one food group. Third graders can then select one or two serving sizes to draw and label for their respective food groups. Now the cafeteria can be a place for *learning* about nutrition too!

Music

School cafeterias are usually busy and chaotic places for eating. Wouldn't it be nice if students could relax, unwind, eat, and talk for twenty minutes each day (or longer!) rather than be placed in a hectic, fast-pace atmosphere? To change the pace and improve the mood of the cafeteria environment, play "mood music" during meals. First, second, and third grade classes can rotate turns each month selecting then playing music from cassette or compact discs in the cafeteria. Who knows, you might even be able to hear the music sometimes!

Across the Curriculum

Introduction to Unit 2 Themes

Now that you've been introduced to the unit by reading *The Edible Pyramid* (Leedy, 1995) and doing nutrition-related activities Across the Curriculum, it is time to study the Food Pyramid in a little more detail. First graders will now learn about the concept of *variety* in the foods that they eat. Second graders will learn about the concept of *moderation* when eating a variety of foods. And third graders will learn how to recognize and measure *serving sizes* for the different food groups.

How Should You Proceed?

The rest of the unit is divided into six focused themes. Six focused themes includes the five different food groups and a sixth category called Fats, Oils, & Sweets. First, second, and third graders will work through each focused theme in sequential order at the rate of approximately one theme per week.

Hence, this unit called "Building the Food Pyramid" may last an additional six weeks. Your local needs and preferences will determine when and how long you will study a Food Group. We do hope you will cover the material in this unit, because the content in these six focused themes serves as a building block to the subsequent units in this book. Without the foundation content in Unit 2, students will not be able to develop the understanding and skills to practice nutrition concepts in different contexts over the course of the school year.

How Are the Focused Themes Organized?

Each focused theme begins with an introductory title page. The title page has two important sections: 1) why the particular food group is important, and 2) examples of foods found in the food group. The title page is followed by the Featured Book for the Unit. In this unit, all of the featured books except for one are non-fiction. This makes this unit unique, because all other units have used fictional picture books to teach food and nutrition concepts.

Why are the Featured Books in each Focused Theme predominately non-fiction books?

A non-fiction book like *A Book of Fruit* (Lember, 1994) is used to introduce the Focused Theme of Fruit Group. A non-fiction book was chosen for all the Focused Themes, except one, because there are many authentic, beautifully photographed books showing real food examples. For the focused theme of Meat, Poultry, Fish, Dry Beans, Eggs, & Nuts Group, no such book exists that encompasses all the various forms of protein. As such, a fictionalized story called *Olson's Meat Pies* (Cohen and Landstrom, 1989) was selected, because we had very few books from which to select a candidate.

What Lesson Plans Accompany Each Focused Theme?

Each Focused Theme will have the Featured Book, followed by three pages of Lesson Plans. The Lesson Plans are designated by grade levels. As stated above, the first grade lesson plans will focus on the concept of *variety*. The second grade lesson plans will focus on the concept of *moderation*. And the third grade lesson plans will focus on the concept of *serving sizes*. You are encouraged to use the Featured Book as a medium for discussing the grade-level concepts. Please use additional books listed in the "Other Books to Read" section to broaden your students understanding of variety, moderation, and serving sizes. The "Other Books to Read" section include both fiction and non-fiction selections. Ideally, all the books will serve as excellent examples for the six Focused Themes.

Focused Theme:
Bread, Cereal, Rice, & Pasta Group

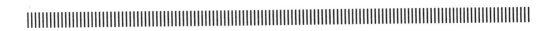

- **Breads, Cereals, Rices, and Pasta are important, because they...**

⇒ are complex carbohydrates which **give us energy for growth and play**.
⇒ **contain vitamins** such as riboflavin, thiamin, and niacin.
⇒ **contain minerals** such as magnesium and iron.
⇒ **add fiber** to our diets.

- **Examples of Breads, Cereals, Rices, and Pastas:**

⇒ bread, rolls, biscuits, and crackers made from grains (corn, wheat, oats, barley, rye, millet, buckwheat, sorghum, bulgur)
⇒ tortillas
⇒ cereals (whole grains, ready-to-eat, and cooked)
⇒ bagels
⇒ rice (white, brown, wild)
⇒ pastas (macaroni, spaghetti, noodles, tortellini)
⇒ sweet corn and popcorn
⇒ pancakes, waffles, and crepes
⇒ muffins, croissants, doughnuts, granola
⇒ potatoes, yams (sweet potatoes), and cassava (tapioca)
NOTE: potatoes, yams (sweet potatoes), and cassava (tapioca) can be counted as vegetables since they are starchy roots, but they are best counted as a bread serving. In this book, potatoes and yams will be counted as vegetable servings. Corn is another confusing food. We can classify corn as a starchy grain and as a frozen or canned vegetable. In this book, corn will be counted as a bread serving.

Featured Book of the Focused Theme: Bread, Cereal, Rice, & Pasta Group	# *Bread, Bread, Bread* # by Ann Morris # Lothrop, Lee & Shepard Books, 1989

This lesson addresses the following Dietary Guidelines for Americans:

⇒ *1. Eat a variety of foods.*
2. Balance the food you eat with physical activity; maintain or improve your weight.
⇒ *3. Choose a diet with plenty of grain products, vegetables, and fruits.*
4. Choose a diet low in fat, saturated fat, and cholesterol.
5. Choose a diet moderate in sugars.
6. Choose a diet moderate in salt and sodium.
7. Choose an alcohol and drug-free lifestyle.

This lesson highlights the following food groups from the Food Guide Pyramid:

⇒ *Bread, Cereal, Rice, & Pasta Group*
Fruit Group
Vegetable Group
Milk, Yogurt, & Cheese Group
Meat, Poultry, Fish, Dry Beans, Eggs, & Nuts Group

Food Guide Pyramid
A Guide to Daily Food Choices

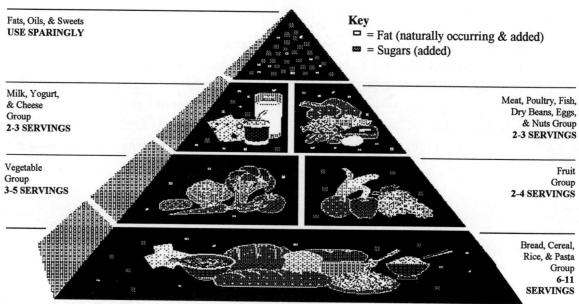

Fats, Oils, & Sweets
USE SPARINGLY

Key
☐ = Fat (naturally occurring & added)
▨ = Sugars (added)

Milk, Yogurt, & Cheese Group
2-3 SERVINGS

Meat, Poultry, Fish, Dry Beans, Eggs, & Nuts Group
2-3 SERVINGS

Vegetable Group
3-5 SERVINGS

Fruit Group
2-4 SERVINGS

Bread, Cereal, Rice, & Pasta Group
6-11 SERVINGS

Source: U.S. Department of Agriculture & U.S. Department of Health and Human Services

Lesson Concept for Grade 1

Important Concepts to Teach about the Bread, Cereal, Rice, & Pasta Group

First Grade Concept — Variety

Bread

Make a list and count the number of different bread choices in the book, *Bread, Bread, Bread.* What grains are found in your favorite type of bread? Rolls? Bagels? Muffins? Buns? Biscuits? What do food labels on bread wrappers tell you about the ingredients in bread and bread products? Can you find wheat bread that is not made with wheat flour? What type of breads do you like for a sandwich? For bread and jelly? What's your favorite bread for toast? For French toast? Do you like bagels with margarine or cream cheese? How many variety of bagels are there in a bagel shop? Did you know that pumpernickle bread is made with rye and potatoes? Do you like rye bread with seeds or without seeds? Do you like cornbread baked like a cake or as muffins? Wow, you can try a variety of grains in a variety of ways with a variety of toppings, spreads, and fillings!

Cereal

Make a list of different breakfast cereals you have eaten. Bring your empty cereal boxes to class when you have eaten all your cereal, so your class can make a long line of cereal boxes across your classroom. How many boxes of each cereal do you have? What cereal wins the top choice for your whole class? Second place? Third place? Are these cereals made with bran, rice, corn, oats, or wheat? Enjoy a small bowl of cereal and milk in class as a snack. Or you can eat cereal right out of the box as a crunchy snack! Cereal is fortified with essential vitamins and minerals, so it is a more healthful snack than chips and snack crackers. While eating your cereal snack, talk about the variety of hot grains that people eat. Have you ever eaten oatmeal? Grits? Hominy?

Rice

On your next visit to the grocery store, notice how rice is sold in different boxes and bags. Make a comparison chart for the rices according to color, shape (long grain or short grain), and length of cooking time. What kind of recipes are on the boxes for the different kinds of rices? What other foods have you eaten that contain rice? Some examples might be rice krispy cereal, rice chex cereal, puffed rice cereal, rice cakes, rice pudding, and rice-a-roni. Did you ever realize there were so many varieties of rice and rice products? Visit an international grocerer to see how rice is sold in bulk and in 20 and 50 pound bags!

Pasta

Pasta comes in many shapes and sizes. Bring an assortment of pasta to class to look at the variety of choices. Sort the different kinds of pasta by spaghetti, ziti, shell macaroni, elbow macaroni, wheel macaroni, bowties, tortellini, ravoli, lasagna, thin noodles, wide noodles, angel hair noodles, couscous, and ramen noodles. You can even categorize pasta by different flavors (tomato, spinach, and egg)! Bring in a favorite recipe using pasta. Talk about a variety of ways to make spaghetti, macaroni and cheese, lasagna, or other dishes. Now that's a lot of pasta!

Lesson Concept for Grade 2

Important Concepts to Teach about the
Bread, Cereal, Rice, & Pasta Group

Second Grade Concept — Moderation

Eat Anytime	Whole-grain breakfast cereals Whole-grain cooked oatmeal or grits Whole-grain or enriched bread Whole-grain or enriched rolls Whole-grain or enriched bagels Whole-grain or enriched tortillas English muffins Low-fat crackers, e.g., graham Brown or enriched white rice Whole-grain or enriched pasta Plain popcorn Pretzels Low-fat cookies, e.g., fig bars Angel food cake
Eat in Moderation	Biscuits Bread stuffing Corn bread Muffins and other quick breads Pancakes Waffles Popcorn made with added fat Taco shells Hushpuppies Dumplings
Eat Occasionally	High-fat crackers Croissants Doughnuts Sweet rolls Snack potato chips Snack corn chips Most cookies Most cakes Most pies

Lesson Concept for Grade 3

Important Concepts to Teach about the Bread, Cereal, Rice, & Pasta Group

Third Grade Concept — Serving Sizes

Recommended Serving Sizes

⇒ **1 slice bread**
⇒ **1 muffin**
⇒ **1 tortilla**
⇒ **1 pancake (4-inch)**
⇒ **3-4 plain crackers (small)**
⇒ **1 ounce ready-to-eat cereal**
⇒ **1/2 cup cooked cereal**
⇒ **1/2 cup pasta**
⇒ **1/2 cup rice**
⇒ **1/2 bagel**
⇒ **1/2 English muffin**
⇒ **1/2 hamburger roll**
⇒ **1/2 croissant (large)**
⇒ **1/2 doughnut (medium)**
⇒ **1/2 danish (medium)**
⇒ **1/16 cake (average)**
⇒ **1/12 pie (2-crust, 8")**
⇒ **2 cookies (medium)**
⇒ **6 pretzels**

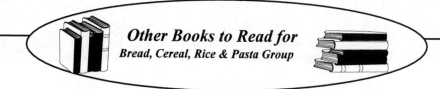

Other Books to Read for
Bread, Cereal, Rice & Pasta Group

This list contains excellent books to read for learning about the Bread, Cereal, Rice & Pasta Group. Use these books along with the Featured Book when teaching the concepts on the previous pages.

Barrett, J. (1978). Cloudy with a chance of meatballs. New York: Scholastic Inc.
> As Grandpa is preparing pancakes for his family, a pancake flies across the room which reminds him of a story. He tells his family about a far away land with strange weather that comes three times a day. Whatever falls from the sky is what everyone eats for that day.

dePaola, T. (1978). The popcorn book. New York: Scholastic Inc.
> Where does popcorn come from? This book gives the history of popcorn along with some helpful hints for storing, preparing, and popping popcorn.

dePaola, T. (1989). Tony's bread. New York: Putnam Publishing Group.
> In order to win the hand of Serafina, Angelo helps Tony the Baker, who is Serafina's father, create the best tasting bread in Milano, Italy. The bread is a success, and Angelo and Serafina marry.

Fowler, A. (1994). Corn-on and off the cob. Chicago: Childrens Press.
> The many different ways corn can be used and prepared are discussed. Other topics include the history of corn and the way corn is grown. (Non-fiction).

Leedy, L. (1994). The edible pyramid: Good eating every day. New York: Holiday House.
> The Edible Pyramid restaurant opens as the maitre d' explains the food pyramid menu to the customers. The maitre d' discusses which foods are included in each group. He also discusses how many servings from each group should be eaten everyday.

Moncure, J. B. (1985). What was it before it was bread? Chicago: Child's World, Inc.
> A loaf of bread begins as a tiny seed from which flour then dough is made. Describes the steps at the bakery and at the grocery store. (Non-fiction).

Sendak, M. (1986). Chicken soup with rice. New York: Scholastic Inc.
> A little boy travels through the months of the year and explains how he would enjoy chicken soup with rice each month.

Shiefman, V. (1994). Sunday potatoes, monday potatoes. New York: Simon & Schuster Books.
> A poor family eats potatoes every day of the week except Saturday. On Saturday, they eat potato pudding.

Other Books to Read, Continued

Turner, D. (1989). <u>Bread</u>. Minneapolis, MN: Carolrhoda Books, Inc.
    A comprehensive look at bread is presented. Topics include the history of bread, the differences between leavened and unleavened bread, the nutritional value of bread, and the different beliefs concerning bread. Recipes for making whole wheat bread and chappatis are given. (Non-fiction).

Watts, B. (1987). <u>Potato</u>. Morristown, NJ: Silver Burdett Press.
    A series of photographs help explain the life of a potato from shoot to tuber. Soon the potato is ready to be dug up and eaten. (Non-fiction).

Wolff, F. (1993). <u>Seven loaves of bread</u>. New York: William Morrow & Co., Inc.
    Milly bakes seven loaves of bread each morning. She shares it with all the barnyard animals. When Milly gets sick, Rose takes over the baking and tries to take some shortcuts. However, she finds out that in the long run, it's easier to bake seven loaves of bread.

Focused Theme: Fruit Group

♦ **Fruits are important, because they...**

⇒ **help our body fight infections** by giving us Vitamin C.
⇒ **help our skin, bones, and eyes stay healthy** by giving us Vitamin A.
⇒ **contain potassium**, an electrolyte, which helps the heart beat properly.
⇒ **add fiber** to our diets.
⇒ **are naturally low in fat, cholesterol, and sodium**.

♦ **Examples of Fruits:**

⇒ apples
⇒ bananas
⇒ oranges
⇒ tangarines
⇒ pears
⇒ peaches
⇒ grapes
⇒ berries (blueberries, raspberries, strawberries, blackberries, cranberries)
⇒ cherries
⇒ grapefruit
⇒ apricots
⇒ plums
⇒ cantaloupe
⇒ honeydew
⇒ dried fruit (dates, raisins, prunes)
⇒ watermelon
⇒ mangos
⇒ starfruit

A Book of Fruit
by Barbara Hirsch Lember
Ticknor & Fields Books for Young
Readers, 1994

This lesson addresses the following Dietary Guidelines for Americans:

⇒   *1. Eat a variety of foods.*
     2. Balance the food you eat with physical activity; maintain or improve your weight.
⇒   *3. Choose a diet with plenty of grain products, vegetables, and fruits.*
     4. Choose a diet low in fat, saturated fat, and cholesterol.
     5. Choose a diet moderate in sugars.
     6. Choose a diet moderate in salt and sodium.
     7. Choose an alcohol and drug-free lifestyle.

This lesson highlights the following food groups from the Food Guide Pyramid:

     Bread, Cereal, Rice, & Pasta Group
⇒   *Fruit Group*
     Vegetable Group
     Milk, Yogurt, & Cheese Group
     Meat, Poultry, Fish, Dry Beans, Eggs, & Nuts Group

Food Guide Pyramid
A Guide to Daily Food Choices

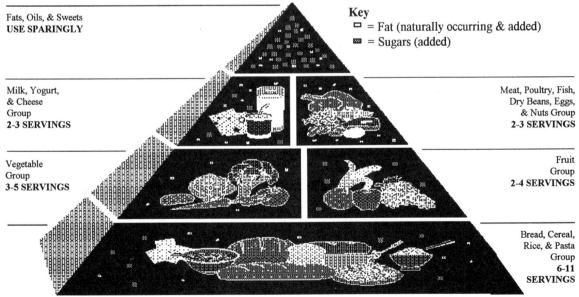

Source: U.S. Department of Agriculture & U.S. Department of Health and Human Services

33

Lesson Concept for Grade 1

Important Concepts to Teach about the Fruit Group

First Grade Concept — Variety

How many varieties of fruits are there? Fruits can be classified as pomes*, drupes*, berries, citrus, tropical, and melons. Use the Featured Book, *A Book of Fruit*, to help you make a list of fruit. What other fruits can you add to your list? What kinds of fruit go into a fruit salad? How many varieties of fruit salads have you eaten? What fruits do you eat on your cereal? In what season(s) do you tend to eat these? Fruits tend to be very seasonal, although worldwide markets make many fruits available year round. Make a list of fruits below that you like to eat during different seasons of the year. Use food props or pictures of fruits to display your class preferences for the current season.

<u>Autumn</u>

<u>Winter</u>

<u>Spring</u>

<u>Summer</u>

*Pomes include apples and pears. Drupes include cherries, peaches, plums, and apricots.

Lesson Concept for Grade 2

Important Concepts to Teach about the Fruit Group

Second Grade Concept — Moderation

Eat Anytime	All fresh fruits All frozen fruits All canned fruits All dried fruits (prunes, dates, figs, raisins, apricots, apples, bananas, etc.) All fruit juices
Eat in Moderation	Fruit juices with added sugar Fruit syrups Sorbets
Eat Occasionally	Fruit pies Fruit jams and jellies

Lesson Concept for Grade 3

Important Concepts to Teach about the Fruit Group

Third Grade Concept — Serving Sizes

Recommended Serving Sizes

⇒ **1 medium fruit (apple, banana, orange)**
⇒ **1/2 grapefruit**
⇒ **1 medium-wedge melon**
⇒ **1/2 cup berries**
⇒ **1/2 cup chopped fruit**
⇒ **1/2 cup canned fruit**
⇒ **1/2 cup cooked fruit**
⇒ **1/4 cup dried fruit**
⇒ **3/4 cup (6 ounces) fruit juice**

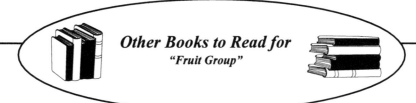

Other Books to Read for
"Fruit Group"

This list contains excellent books to read for learning about the Fruit Group. Use these books along with the featured book when teaching the concepts on the previous pages.

Barrett, J. (1978). Cloudy with a chance of meatballs. New York: Scholastic Inc.
    As Grandpa is preparing pancakes for his family, a pancake flies across the room which reminds him of a story. He tells his family about a far away land with strange weather that comes three times a day. Whatever falls from the sky is what everyone eats for that day.

Coldrey, J., & Bernard, G. (1988). Strawberry. Englewood Cliffs, NJ: Silver Burdett Press.
    A series of photographs show the life of a strawberry from seedling to pollinization. They are soon ripe enough to be eaten by people and animals. (Non-fiction).

Cole, S. (1991). When the rain stops. New York: Lothrop, Lee and Shepard Books.
    Beautiful illustrations show a little girl, her dad, and several animals prepare for a rainstorm. After the rain stops, the animals come out of their shelters, and the girl and her dad go back outside to pick blueberries.

Darling, B. (1992). Valerie and the silver pear. New York: Macmillan Children's Book Group.
    Valerie enjoys visiting her grandfather. One day, during her visit, he tells her a story of a pear tree. After hearing the story, they decide to make pear pies.

Day, J. W. (1976). What is a fruit? New York: Golden Press.
    Children learn what makes a particular food a fruit. Traditional fruits such as apples, oranges, and bananas are featured. Foods that are not commonly thought of as fruit such as walnuts, almonds, tomatoes, cucumbers, peas, grains of corn, and grains of rice are also featured. (Non-fiction).

Degen, B. (1985). Jamberry. New York: Scholastic Inc.
    A boy and his bear friend love berries. They rhyme about berry picking while walking in the forest and decide what they are going to do with their berries.

Ehlert, L. (1993). Eating the alphabet: Fruits and vegetables from a to z. San Diego: Harcourt Brace.
    There are fruits and vegetables from A-Z. A is for apple, asparagus, avocado, apricot and artichoke. B is for brussel sprouts, bean, blueberry, broccoli and banana.

Other Books to Read,
Continued

Fowler, A. (1994). Apples of your eye. Chicago: Childrens Press.
> The different types of apples and their by-products are discussed. Children will learn about grafting in order to produce good apples and the type of environment needed to grow apples. (Non-fiction).

Joosse, B. M. (1987). Jam day. New York: HarperCollins Children's Books.
> An annual family reunion involving berry picking and jam making reminds Ben that he is part of a big family, even though his immediate family is small. It is a noisy family of grandparents, cousins, uncles, and aunts.

Kindersley, D. (1991). My first look at shopping. New York: Random House, Inc.
> There are many things people can buy when they go shopping. At the grocery, there are apples, oranges, peppers, grapes, bananas, corn and lemons. At the bakery, there are cakes, croissants, fruit tarts, bread and pastries. There are many other stores to visit too.

Lapp, E. (1983). The blueberry bears. Niles, IL: Albert Whitman & Company.
> Bessie loves to pick blueberries in the woods behind her house. She picks so many blueberries that every container is filled. The bears go to Bessie's house to eat her blueberries because she picked all of the blueberries in the woods!

Leedy, L. (1994). The edible pyramid: Good eating every day. New York: Holiday House.
> The Edible Pyramid restaurant opens as the maitre d' explains the food pyramid menu to the customers. The maitre d' discusses which foods are included in each group. He also discusses how many servings from each group should be eaten everyday.

McCloskey, R. (1976). Blueberries for sal. New York: Scholastic Inc.
> Little Sal picks blueberries with her mom then wanders off. She finds a bear who is looking for her baby. The bear and Sal wander around together to help the bear find her baby and Sal find her mom.

Micucci, C. (1992). The life and the times of the apple. New York: Orchard Books.
> A comprehensive look at many aspects of the apple is described. Topics include the life of the apple, the history of the apple, the different uses of the apple, and the different varieties of apples. (Non-fiction).

Moncure, J. B. (1985). What was it before it was orange juice? Chicago: Child's World, Inc.
> A boy asks his mother, "What was orange juice before it was orange juice?" Describes how orange juice starts as a tiny seed. The tiny seed then grows into an orange tree and is eventually manufactured into juice. (Non-fiction).

*Other Books to Read,
Continued*

McGuire, R. (1994). The orange book. New York: Puffin Books.
   Fourteen oranges grow on a tree. Many different things happen to these oranges. Some become a snack, some are used in a juggling act, and others are made into juice.

McMillan, B. (1986). Becca backwards, becca frontwards: A book of concept pairs. New York: Lothrop, Lee and Shepard Books.
   Through the use of photographs, a little girl named Becca, displays opposites. For example, a full glass of milk and an empty glass of milk are opposites.

McMillan, B. (1991). Eating fractions. New York: Scholastic Inc.
   Using foods like muffins and pizza, two children divide up and share food in three quantities (one-half, one-third and one-fourth).

McMillan, B. (1988). Growing colors. New York: Lothrup, Lee and Shepard Books.
   Fruits and vegetables illustrate a rainbow of colors.

Munz, E. (1975). Happily appley. New York: Girl Scouts of the U.S.A.
   A comprehensive look at apples is presented. Items include recipes (apple egg nog, applesauce-raisin bread, Johnny Appleseed meatballs), activities (fruit and vegetable prints and apple head dolls), apple lore, how apples are grown, and the different varieties of apples. (Non-fiction).

Nottridge, R. (1991). Apples. Minneapolis, MN: Carolrhoda Books, Inc.
   A comprehensive look at apples is presented. Topics include growing apples, making apple cider, and the history of the apple and Johnny Appleseed. (Non-fiction).

Robinson, F. (1992). We love fruit! Chicago: Childrens Press.
   Different types of fruit are shown and what makes a food a fruit. (Non-fiction).

Schaefer, J. J. (1994). Miranda's day to dance. New York: Macmillan Children's Book Group.
   Miranda collects tropical fruit each day of the week in order to make a headdress to wear on Sunday, which is her day to dance. Fruits such as bananas, pineapples, and raspberries are shown with a different animal indigenous to South America.

Watts, B. (1989). Tomato. Englewood Cliffs, NJ: Silver Burdett Press.
   A series of photographs help explain the life of a tomato from seed to pollinization to being ripe enough to be picked off the vine. (Non-fiction).

Focused Theme: Vegetable Group

||||||||||||||||||||||||||||||||||||||||||||||||||||||||||||||||||||||||||||||||||||||||||||||||||||

- ◆ **Vegetables are important, because they...**
  ⇒ **help our skin, bones, and eyes stay healthy** by giving us Vitamin A.
  ⇒ **help our body fight off germs** by giving us Vitamin C.
  ⇒ **contain minerals** such as potassium and magnesium.
  ⇒ **add fiber to our diets.**
  ⇒ **are naturally low in fat and cholesterol.**

- ◆ **Examples of Vegetables:**
  ⇒ broccoli
  ⇒ cauliflower
  ⇒ celery
  ⇒ lettuce (leaf, iceberg, romaine, Boston, bibb, Belgian endive, curly endive)
  ⇒ leafy greens (spinach, mustard greens, kale (collard greens), turnip greens, sorrel, broccoli rapini, arugula, radicchio)
  ⇒ cabbage (including bok choy)
  ⇒ carrots
  ⇒ green beans
  ⇒ peas (green peas, snap peas, Oriental peas, split peas)
  ⇒ brussel sprouts
  ⇒ bean sprouts
  ⇒ mushrooms
  ⇒ tomatoes
  ⇒ pumpkins
  ⇒ cucumbers and radishes
  ⇒ squash (acorn, butternut, zucchini, spaghetti)
  ⇒ peppers (green bell peppers, red sweet peppers, yellow banana peppers)
  ⇒ okra
  ⇒ onions (sweet, green, vandalia, leeks)
  ⇒ potatoes and yams (sweet potatoes) (NOTE: potatoes, yams, and cassava (tapioca) can be counted as vegetables since they are starchy roots, but they are often counted as a bread serving. In this book, potatoes and yams will be counted as vegetable servings. Corn is another confusing food. We can classify corn as a starchy grain and as a frozen or canned vegetable. In this book, corn will be counted as a bread serving.)

<table>
<tr><td>

Featured Book
of the Focused Theme:
Vegetable Group

</td><td>

Vegetable in the Garden
by Pascale de Bourgoing and
Gallimard Jeunesse
Scholastic Inc., 1989

</td></tr>
</table>

This lesson addresses the following Dietary Guidelines for Americans:

⇒   *1. Eat a variety of foods.*

     2. Balance the food you eat with physical activity; maintain or improve your weight.

⇒   *3. Choose a diet with plenty of grain products, vegetables, and fruits.*

     4. Choose a diet low in fat, saturated fat, and cholesterol.

     5. Choose a diet moderate in sugars.

     6. Choose a diet moderate in salt and sodium.

     7. Choose an alcohol and drug-free lifestyle.

This lesson highlights the following food groups from the Food Guide Pyramid:

     Bread, Cereal, Rice, & Pasta Group

     Fruit Group

⇒   *Vegetable Group*

     Milk, Yogurt, & Cheese Group

     Meat, Poultry, Fish, Dry Beans, Eggs, & Nuts Group

Food Guide Pyramid
A Guide to Daily Food Choices

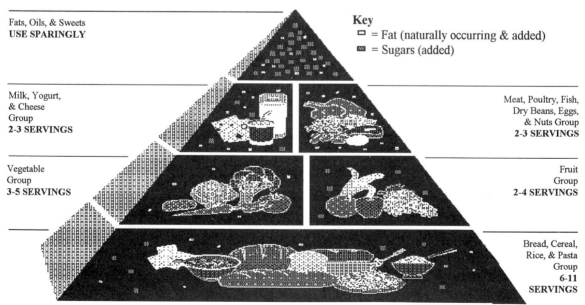

Source: U.S. Department of Agriculture & U.S. Department of Health and Human Services

Lesson Concept for Grade 1

Important Concepts to Teach about the Vegetable Group

First Grade Concept — Variety

There are many varieties of vegetables. A variety of vegetables can be classified by their color. Did you know that orange, yellow, and red vegetables are especially rich in Vitamin A? Did you know that all vegetables contain Vitamin C? How many variety of vegetables have you eaten? Not eaten? How many of these vegetables would you be willing to try? Are there some vegetables that you prefer to eat raw? Cooked? Draw or cut out pictures of colorful vegetables and make a vegetable rainbow on your classroom wall. You might even visit a farmer's market or greengrocer in your community and observe their rainbows of colorful vegetables row after row.

Green vegetables: broccoli, celery, lettuce, leafy greens, cabbage, green beans, peas, brussel sprouts, cucumbers, peppers, asparagus, okra

Red vegetables: tomatoes, peppers

Yellow vegetables: squash, onions, potatoes, peppers

Orange vegetables: carrots, pumpkins, yams (sweet potatoes), peppers

White vegetables: cauliflower, bean sprouts, mushrooms, radishes, onions, potatoes, turnips

Purple vegetables: eggplant

In addition to color varieties, vegetables can be classified by type. Can you add to the list below?

Seeds: corn, peas

Roots: sweet potato, carrot, beet, radish, turnip, potato

Stalks: asparagus, celery, mushroom, rhubarb

Leaves: cabbage, lettuce, parsley, spinach

Flowers: broccoli, cauliflower

Fruits: banana squash, cucumber, pepper, pumpkin, tomato, zucchini

Lesson Concept for Grade 2

Important Concepts to Teach about the Vegetable Group

Second Grade Concept — Moderation

Eat Anytime	All fresh vegetables, except corn All frozen vegetables, except corn All canned vegetables, except corn All vegetable juices Plain potato Potato with low-fat topping Tomato sauces
Eat in Moderation	Vegetables with added margarine Vegetables with added butter Potatoes topped with butter Potatoes topped with sour cream Potatoes topped with sauces Mashed potatoes Hash brown potatoes
Eat Occasionally	Deep-fried vegetables French fries Vegetables in cream sauce Vegetables in cheese sauce

Lesson Concept for Grade 3

Important Concepts to Teach about the Vegetable Group

Third Grade Concept — Serving Sizes

Recommended Serving Sizes

⇒ **1 cup of raw leafy vegetables**
⇒ **1/2 cup of cooked vegetables**
⇒ **1/2 cup of chopped raw vegetables**
⇒ **3/4 cup (6 ounces) vegetable juice**
⇒ **1 medium potato or yam**
⇒ **1/2 cup scalloped potatoes**
⇒ **1/2 cup potato salad**

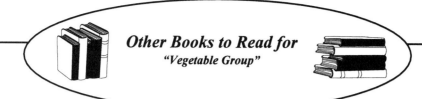

Other Books to Read for
"Vegetable Group"

This list contains excellent books to read for learning about the Vegetable Group. Use these books along with the Featured Book when teaching the concepts on the previous pages.

Barrett, J. (1978). Cloudy with a chance of meatballs. New York: Scholastic Inc.
> As Grandpa is preparing pancakes for his family, a pancake flies across the room which reminds him of a story. He tells his family about a far away land with strange weather that comes three times a day. Whatever falls from the sky is what everyone eats for that day.

Brown, M. (1947). Stone soup. New York: Aladdin Books.
> Three hungry soldiers walk down the road. They stop at several houses to ask for food, but nobody has any extra to share. One of the soldiers tricks the townspeople and says he can make stone soup. By the time the soup is finished, all of the townspeople contribute some type of food to the soup.

Ehlert, L. (1993). Eating the alphabet: Fruits and vegetables from a to z. San Diego: Harcourt Brace
> There are fruits and vegetables from A-Z. A is for apple, asparagus, avocado, apricot and artichoke. B is for brussel sprouts, bean, blueberry, broccoli and banana.

Ehlert, L. (1990). Growing vegetable soup. San Diego: Scholastic Inc.
> Shows the process of planting, growing, and eating colorful vegetables for soup.

Gage, W. (1976). Squash pie. New York: Greenwillow Books.
> Due to his love for squash pie, a farmer plants many crops of squash, only to have them stolen repeatedly. The farmer creates different devices to catch the thief, but fails on each attempt. His wife admits to the crime and discovers her own love for squash pies.

Harper, J. (1993). Jalapeno hal. New York: Macmillan Children's Book Group.
> Jalapeno Hal is a cowboy who is the roughest and toughest man in all of Texas. Hal and his friend Kit have a plan to get the whole town hopping.

King, C. (1994). The vegetables go to bed. New York: Crown Publishers.
> The vegetables are going to bed. Lettuce, peas, carrots, cabbage, beans, tomatoes, and corn are tucked in for the night. When the sun goes down, it is bedtime for the vegetables and also for you!

Other Books to Read,
Continued

Leedy, L. (1994). <u>The edible pyramid</u>: <u>Good eating every day</u>. New York: Holiday House.
  The Edible Pyramid restaurant opens as the maitre d' explains the food pyramid menu to the customers. The maitre d' discusses which foods are included in each group. He also discusses how many servings from each group should be eaten everyday.

McMillan, B. (1988). <u>Growing colors</u>. New York: Lothrup, Lee and Shepard Books.
  Fruits and vegetables illustrate a rainbow of colors.

McNulty, F. (1987). <u>The lady and the spider</u>. New York: HarperCollins Children's Books.
  A spider lives peacefully in a head of lettuce in a lady's garden. The lady sees the spider when she cleans the lettuce and returns the spider to the garden.

Robinson, F. (1994). <u>Vegetables, vegetables</u>! Chicago: Childrens Press.
  Photographs show that vegetables come from leaves, roots, or flowers of certain plants. Differences between a fruit and a vegetable are shown, and how vegetables can be eaten or prepared by themselves or with other foods. (Non-fiction).

Steele, M. (1989). <u>Anna's garden songs</u>. New York: Scholastic Inc.
  Anna spends the day in her garden. She picks beets, potatoes, rhubarb, radishes, lettuce, carrots, peas, tomatoes, cherries, onions, cabbage, leek, herbs, and nasturtium. Anna likes to sing as she picks her vegetables.

Focused Theme:
Milk, Yogurt, & Cheese Group

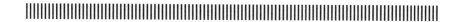

♦ **Milk, Yogurt, and Cheeses are important, because they...**

⇒ **keep our bones and teeth strong, and help our muscles move** by giving us calcium.
⇒ **help our bones and teeth grow** by giving us Vitamin D.
⇒ **help our skin, bones, and eyes stay healthy** by giving us Vitamin A and riboflavin.

♦ **Examples of Milk Products:**

⇒ milk (skim, 1/2%, 1%, 2%, whole, chocolate, buttermilk, fortified soy-milk)
⇒ yogurt, including frozen yogurt
⇒ yellow cheese (colby, cheddar, cojack)
⇒ white cheese (mozarella, munster, swiss,)
⇒ ice cream, ice milk, and sherbet
⇒ cream
⇒ sour cream
⇒ cream cheese
⇒ cottage cheese
⇒ custard and puddings

Featured Book of the Focused Theme: Milk, Yogurt, & Cheese Group

Milk from Cow to Carton
by Aliki
HarperCollins Publishers, 1992

This lesson addresses the following Dietary Guidelines for Americans:

1. Eat a variety of foods.
2. Balance the food you eat with physical activity; maintain or improve your weight.
3. Choose a diet with plenty of grain products, vegetables, and fruits.
⇒ 4. *Choose a diet low in fat, saturated fat, and cholesterol.*
5. Choose a diet moderate in sugars.
6. Choose a diet moderate in salt and sodium.
7. Choose an alcohol and drug-free lifestyle.

This lesson highlights the following food groups from the Food Guide Pyramid:

Bread, Cereal, Rice, & Pasta Group

Fruit Group

Vegetable Group

⇒ *Milk, Yogurt, & Cheese Group*

Meat, Poultry, Fish, Dry Beans, Eggs, & Nuts Group

Food Guide Pyramid
A Guide to Daily Food Choices

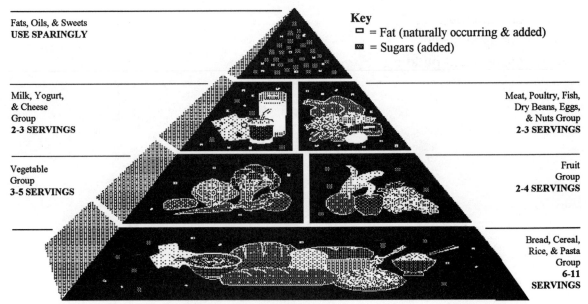

Source: U.S. Department of Agriculture & U.S. Department of Health and Human Services

Lesson Concept for Grade 1

Important Concepts to Teach about the
Milk, Yogurt, & Cheese Group

First Grade Concept — Variety

Milk

Go for variety when you take a drink! After water, milk should be your number one choice for a drink. Milk comes in three flavors (white, chocolate, and strawberry) and has a variety of compositions. Do you like skim milk, 1/2 percent milk, 1 percent milk, or 2 percent milk? Young babies under two years of age drink homogenized whole milk or 2 percent milk for the extra fat calories to help them grow. Infants under one year of age drink breast milk or formula milk. And there's even many different types and varieties of formula milk! The most nutritious milk in town is skim milk. Skim milk is lowest in fat and highest in calcium which is the mineral that makes your bones grow. Foods like pudding, which is made with milk, is another clever way of getting enough of your daily serving size. Now that's a fun variety of milk! What does your family make with buttermilk? Pancakes? Bread? Muffins? Does anyone in your family drink acidophilus milk? Why? More milk varieties for a variety of people!

Yogurt

There is basic yogurt, vanilla yogurt, fruit-filled yogurt, and crunchy yogurt. There is regular yogurt, lowfat yogurt, and nonfat yogurt. You can buy yogurt in small, medium, and large containers. Frozen yogurt comes in multiple flavors. Do you eat your frozen yogurt in a cup, dish, or cone? How many flavors can you buy? Which yogurts *will* you buy and try? Yogurt is another good way to get calcium in your diet so your bones and teeth can be stronger over your lifetime.

Cheese

Cheese is also made from milk, so enjoy some cheese for a little variety in your diet. Cheese comes in a variety of colors. There are many different white cheeses and many different yellow cheeses. Which cheese is both yellow and white? Cojack, you're right! Choose your cheese by the slice, shredded, or chunked. You can also buy cheese from a carton (cottage cheese or cream cheese), cheese from a jar (cheese spread), and cheese from a box (processed cheese or cream cheese). Swiss cheese has holes in it?! You will never grow bored eating cheese! And when you get older, you'll probably like to try some Brie (France) or Camembert (Normandy) or Stilton (England) cheese. When you consider all the different countries where cheeses are made, there is quite a variety from which to choose. For starters, why don't you choose your favorite three domestic cheeses? Will you eat your cheese on crackers, sprinkled and melted on top of a pizza, baked inside a casserole, or just by itself? Mmmm!

Lesson Concept for Grade 2

Important Concepts to Teach about the
Milk, Yogurt, & Cheese Group

Second Grade Concept — Moderation

Eat Anytime	Skim milk 1% low-fat milk Low-fat buttermilk Plain non-fat yogurt Low-fat yogurt Low-fat cheeses
Eat in Moderation	2% low-fat milk Part skim-milk cheese Ice milk
Eat Occasionally	Whole milk, cream, half-and-half Whole-milk yogurt All regular cheese such as Cheddar, American, Brie, and others Ice cream Cream cheese Sour cream

Lesson Concept for Grade 3

Important Concepts to Teach about the Milk, Yogurt, & Cheese Group

Third Grade Concept — Serving Sizes

Recommended Serving Sizes

⇒ **1 cup (8 ounces) milk**
⇒ **1 cup (8 ounces) yogurt**
⇒ **1.5 ounces natural cheese**
⇒ **2 ounces processed cheese**
⇒ **2 cups cottage cheese**
⇒ **1 cup pudding**
⇒ **1 cup frozen yogurt**
⇒ **1.5 cups ice cream**
⇒ **1.5 cups ice milk**

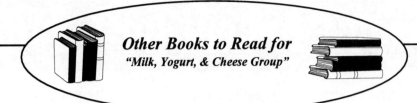

Other Books to Read for
"Milk, Yogurt, & Cheese Group"

This list contains excellent books to read for learning about the Milk, Yogurt, & Cheese Group.
Use these books along with the Featured Book when teaching the concepts on the previous pages.

Barrett, J. (1978). <u>Cloudy with a chance of meatballs</u>. New York: Scholastic Inc.
    As Grandpa is preparing pancakes for his family, a pancake flies across the room which reminds
    him of a story. He tells his family about a far away land with strange weather that comes three
    times a day. Whatever falls from the sky is what everyone eats for that day.

Carrick, D. (1985). <u>Milk</u>. New York: Greenwillow Books.
    This is a behind-the-scene story about milk. It all starts with the cows, and they must be well
    fed. After they eat, the cows are hooked up to the milking machine. When they have been
    milked, the milk truck comes to take away the milk to clean it and make it ready to drink.
    (Non-fiction).

Ericsson, J. (1993). <u>No milk</u>! New York: William Morrow & Co., Inc.
    A little city boy tells jokes, juggles, and sings so a cow will give milk. Eventually, he learns that
    in order to get milk he needs to squeeze the cow's udders.

Leedy, L. (1994). <u>The edible pyramid</u>: <u>Good eating every day</u>. New York: Holiday House.
    The Edible Pyramid restaurant opens as the maitre d' explains the food pyramid menu to the
    customers. The maitre d' discusses which foods are included in each group. He also discusses
    how many servings from each group should be eaten everyday.

Focused Theme: Meat, Poultry, Fish, Dry Beans, Eggs, & Nuts Group

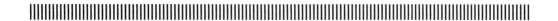

♦ **Meat, Poultry, Fish, Dry, Beans, Eggs, and Nuts are important, because they...**

⇒ are proteins which **help our muscles grow and become stronger.**

⇒ **help our blood use and carry oxygen** throughout our body by giving us iron.

⇒ **help us grow, fight infections, heal wounds, and improves our taste and smell** by giving us zinc.

♦ **Examples of Protein Foods:**

⇒ meat (beef, pork, lamb)

⇒ poultry (chicken, turkey)

⇒ fish

⇒ eggs

⇒ dry beans or legumes (baked beans, kidney beans, navy beans, pinto beans, garbonzo beans, chick peas, refried beans)

⇒ nuts (peanuts, walnuts, pecans, almonds, hazelnuts, chestnuts, pinenuts)

⇒ seeds (pumpkin, sunflower)

*Featured Book
of the Focused Theme:
Meat, Poultry, Fish,
Dry Beans, Eggs, & Nuts
Group*

Olson's Meat Pies
by Peter Cohen & Olof Lanstrom
R & S Books, 1989

This lesson addresses the following Dietary Guidelines for Americans:

1. Eat a variety of foods.
2. Balance the food you eat with physical activity; maintain or improve your weight.
3. Choose a diet with plenty of grain products, vegetables, and fruits.
⇒ *4. Choose a diet low in fat, saturated fat, and cholesterol.*
5. Choose a diet moderate in sugars.
6. Choose a diet moderate in salt and sodium.
7. Choose an alcohol and drug-free lifestyle.

This lesson highlights the following food groups from the Food Guide Pyramid:

Bread, Cereal, Rice, & Pasta Group
Fruit Group
⇒ *Vegetable Group*
Milk, Yogurt, & Cheese Group
⇒ *Meat, Poultry, Fish, Dry Beans, Eggs, & Nuts Group*

Food Guide Pyramid
A Guide to Daily Food Choices

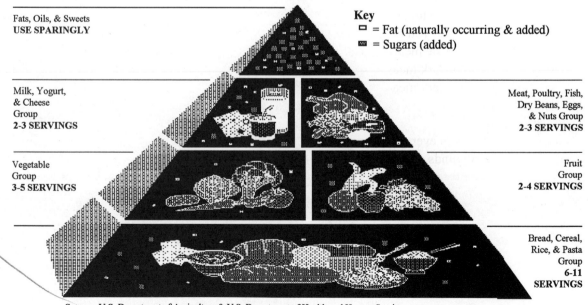

Fats, Oils, & Sweets
USE SPARINGLY

Key
◻ = Fat (naturally occurring & added)
▨ = Sugars (added)

Milk, Yogurt,
& Cheese
Group
2-3 SERVINGS

Meat, Poultry, Fish,
Dry Beans, Eggs,
& Nuts Group
2-3 SERVINGS

Vegetable
Group
3-5 SERVINGS

Fruit
Group
2-4 SERVINGS

Bread, Cereal,
Rice, & Pasta
Group
**6-11
SERVINGS**

Source: U.S. Department of Agriculture & U.S. Department of Health and Human Services

Lesson Concept for Grade 1

Important Concepts to Teach about the
Meat, Poultry, Fish, Dry Beans, Eggs, & Nuts Group

First Grade Concept — Variety

Meat There are so many kinds of meats! There is beef from cattle, lamb from sheep, and pork from pigs. Ham, bacon, and sausage come from pigs too. Sometimes we refer to different meat by the way a butcher cuts it or prepares it. Did you know that hamburger is really beef? The technical word for hamburger is ground beef or ground round or ground chuck depending upon what part of the cattle is used. You also can have ground pork from pigs! Some people even make ground venison from deer. Do you like eating roasts, steaks, chops, or ribs? You can eat roast beef, roast pork, roast lamb, or roast venison. You can also eat chops from pork or lamb. Ribs can be made from beef or pork. Steaks can also be made from beef or pork. Are you confused? Just remember to first decide upon the kind of meat you want to eat, i.e., beef, lamb, pork, or venison. Then figure out what cut or type of meat you want, i.e., ground, roast, steak, chops, or ribs. Wow, we haven't even talked about luncheon meats, beef jerky, kielbasa, or hotdogs?! Maybe you should visit a butcher and ask lots of questions!

Poultry Poultry are domestic birds raised for meat or eggs. Let's talk about the meat in this category and save the eggs for the category below. Do you like chicken, turkey, duck, or goose meat the best? Duck and goose meat? Yes, some people still eat roast duck or roast goose for special holidays, but most people prefer turkey and chicken. What part of the bird do you like best? The drumstick, the thigh, the breast, or the back? Do you prefer white meat or dark meat? Did you know that the white meat of poultry has less fat than the dark meat of poultry? That's why the white meat can sometimes dry out faster than the dark meat if it gets overcooked.

Fish Have you ever gone to a fish fry? Mmmm! Mmm! People all over the world eat so many kinds of fish. What kind of fish have you eaten? Do you like shellfish like crabs and lobster? Fresh fish is stored on ice until its ready to be fried, baked, or grilled. You can buy a whole salmon at the market and cut it into steaks for the grill. Or you can buy salmon in a can and make salmon patties to fry in a pan. What other fish have you eaten from a can? Tuna? Mackerel? What fish have you eaten from a jar? Herring? If you study across the world about the different kinds of fish to eat and the ways to prepare it then eat it, you would be completely amazed. Better start your research! Or go to a local pond, lake, or river to catch a fish for dinner!

Lesson Concept for Grade 1, *cont.*

Important Concepts to Teach about the
Meat, Poultry, Fish, Dry Beans, Eggs, & Nuts Group

First Grade Concept — Variety
Continued

Dry Beans   Another word for dry beans is legumes. If you read about legumes in the dictionary, you would find that there are many plants that fit into this category, including herbs, shrubs, and trees. Wow! Well, for our purposes, let's focus on some more typical legumes that we eat like navy beans, pinto beans, baked beans, kidney beans, red beans, garbonzo beans, split peas, and chick peas. Can you think of any more? Legumes are important in our diets for protein and fiber, so eat some dry beans today!

Eggs   Eggs from chickens, ducks, and geese come in many sizes. How are chicken eggs packaged by size in the dairy case of the grocery store? What do you know about white eggs and brown eggs? Have you ever eaten a large goose egg? The inside yolk is really large. Sometimes you even get a double yolk inside. Eggs are needed for baking cakes, cookies, brownies, muffins, nutbreads, meringues, and other foods like pancakes, waffles, and French toast. You can also cook eggs for breakfast, lunch, or dinner as an omelet, a poached egg, fried egg, scrambled eggs, and hard-boiled eggs. Take your pick! There is plenty of variety in a simple, oval egg!

Nuts   How many different nuts or seeds have you eaten? Let's see, there are almonds, brazil nuts, cashew nuts, chestnuts, coconut, filberts (hazelnuts), macadamia nuts, mixed nuts, peanuts, pecans, pine nuts, pistachio nuts, pumpkin seeds, sesame seeds, sunflower seeds, and walnuts. You can eat them raw or in salads or in pasta, cakes, cookies, muffins, and more! For even more variety, you can choose between dry roasted, oil roasted, honey roasted, shelled, salted, or unsalted. What's your favorite nut or seed to eat? Have you ever bought nuts or seeds in the bulk foods section of the grocery store? Or do you prefer to buy them in a can, jar, or bag?

Lesson Concept for Grade 2

Important Concept to Teach about the
Meat, Poultry, Fish, Dry Beans, Eggs, & Nuts Group

Second Grade Concept — Moderation

Eat Anytime	Lean beef including round, sirloin, chuck, and loin Lean pork cuts including ham and tenderloin Lamb: leg, arm, loin, rib All poultry without skin All fresh and frozen fish Egg whites All beans, peas, and lentils
Eat in Moderation	All poultry with skin Most cuts of beef including all ground beef, short ribs, corned beef brisket Most cuts of pork including chops and loin roast All luncheon meats Peanut butter and other nuts and seeds Eggs limited to three per week
Eat Occasionally	USDA prime-grade cuts of beef Pork spareribs and ground pork Ground lamb Fried fish Sausage Frankfurters Bacon

Lesson Concept for Grade 3

Important Concepts to Teach about the
Meat, Poultry, Fish, Dry Beans, Eggs, & Nuts Group

Third Grade Concept — Serving Sizes

Recommended Serving Sizes

⇒ **2 to 3 ounces of cooked lean beef, pork, lamb, veal, poultry or fish. A 3-ounce piece of meat is about the size of a deck of playing cards.**

⇒ **Count the following as 1 ounce of meat:**
   1 egg
   3 egg whites
   2 tablespoons of peanut butter
   2 tablespoons of whole nuts or seeds
   1/2 cup cooked beans, peas or lentils

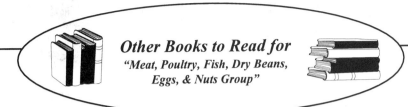

Other Books to Read for
*"Meat, Poultry, Fish, Dry Beans,
Eggs, & Nuts Group"*

This list contains excellent books to read for learning about the Meat, Poultry, Fish, Dry Beans, & Nuts Group. Use these books along with the Featured Book when teaching the concepts on the previous pages.

Barrett, J. (1978). <u>Cloudy with a chance of meatballs</u>. New York: Scholastic Inc.
> As Grandpa is preparing pancakes for his family, a pancake flies across the room which reminds him of a story. He tells his family about a far away land with strange weather that comes three times a day. Whatever falls from the sky is what everyone eats for that day.

Brown, M. (1951). <u>Skipper john's cook</u>. New York: Charles Scribner's Sons.
> A new cook is hired on a ship, because the old cook just fixed beans. After a few days, the crew finds out all the new cook does is fry fish and make beans. Once again, the crew looks for a new cook.

Brown, M. (1947). <u>Stone soup</u>. New York: Aladdin Books.
> Three hungry soldiers walk down the road. They stop at several houses to ask for food, but nobody has any extra to share. One of the soldiers tricks the townspeople and says he can make stone soup. By the time the soup is finished, all of the townspeople contribute some type of food to the soup.

Hammerstein, O. (1992). <u>A real nice clambake</u>. New York: Little, Brown & Co.
> A bunch of friends gather to have a big clambake at the beach. Everyone eats a lot and enjoys the beautiful day.

Leedy, L. (1994). <u>The edible pyramid</u>: <u>Good eating every day</u>. New York: Holiday House.
> The Edible Pyramid restaurant opens as the maitre d' explains the food pyramid menu to the customers. The maitre d' discusses which foods are included in each group. He also discusses how many servings from each group should be eaten everyday.

LeGuin, U. K. (1992). <u>Fish soup</u>. New York: Atheneum Books for Young Readers.
> The thinking man and the writing woman are good friends. They decide to find a child to run messages between their homes and to catch fish for their fish soup. The child is created by their imaginations and a touch of magic.

McCloskey, R. (1976). <u>One morning in maine</u>. New York: Puffin Books.
> Sal and her father goes to the beach to search for clams. During the day, Sal loses her tooth in the mud. She does not cry because she knows that when she looses a tooth she is starting to grow up. They take a boat trip to a nearby island to celebrate with ice cream cones.

Other Books to Read,
Continued

Otey, M. (1993). <u>Blue moon soup spoon</u>. New York: Farrar, Straus & Giroux.
    A boy looks out the window at a blue moon while his mom makes stew. The boy goes outside
    to wait for his dad to come home for dinner. When his dad gets home, they all sit down for
    dinner and the boy eats with his blue moon soup spoon.

Saunders, S. (1982). <u>Fish fry</u>. New York: Puffin Books.
    Edith wakes up and rushes out of bed. She is excited because today is the fish fry. The whole
    town gathers down by the river to fish and have a picnic.

Westcott, N. B. (1992). <u>Peanut butter and jelly</u>. New York: Puffin Books.
    Through a rhyme, two little children show how to make a peanut butter and jelly sandwich.

Focused Theme:
Fats, Oils, & Sweets Group

||||||||||||||||||||||||||||||||||||||||||||||||||||||||||||||||||||||||||||||||||||||||||||||||||

♦ **Fats, Oils, and Sweets should be used sparingly, because they...**

⇒ **contain little or no vitamins and minerals.**
⇒ **increase your chance of becoming overweight.**
⇒ **increase your chance of getting certain diseases as you get older.**

♦ **Examples of Foods with Fats, Oils, and Sweets:**

FATS
⇒ margarine
⇒ salad dressings
⇒ oils
⇒ mayonnaise
⇒ butter
⇒ gravy
⇒ sauces
⇒ shortening

SWEETS
⇒ cake
⇒ pie
⇒ cookies
⇒ doughnuts
⇒ sweet rolls
⇒ candy
⇒ soft drinks
⇒ fruit drinks
⇒ jelly and jam
⇒ syrup
⇒ gelatin
⇒ desserts
⇒ sugar (white sugar, raw sugar, brown sugar, corn syrup, honey, molasses)

| *Featured Book of the Focused Theme: Fats, Oils, & Sweets Group* | ***Chocolate Chip Cookies* by Karen Wagner Henry Holt & Company, 1990** |

This lesson addresses the following Dietary Guidelines for Americans:

1. Eat a variety of foods.
2. Balance the food you eat with physical activity; maintain or improve your weight.
3. Choose a diet with plenty of grain products, vegetables, and fruits.
⇒ 4. *Choose a diet low in fat, saturated fat, and cholesterol.*
⇒ 5. *Choose a diet moderate in sugars.*
6. Choose a diet moderate in salt and sodium.
7. Choose an alcohol and drug-free lifestyle.

This lesson highlights the following food groups from the Food Guide Pyramid:

Bread, Cereal, Rice, & Pasta Group
Fruit Group
Vegetable Group
Milk, Yogurt, & Cheese Group
Meat, Poultry, Fish, Dry Beans, Eggs, & Nuts Group
⇒ *Fats, Oils, & Sweets*

Food Guide Pyramid
A Guide to Daily Food Choices

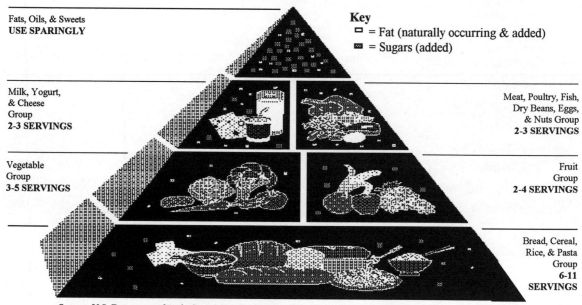

Source: U.S. Department of Agriculture & U.S. Department of Health and Human Services

Lesson Concept for Grade 1

Important Concepts to Teach about the
Fats, Oils, & Sweets Group

First Grade Concept — Variety

Fats and Oils

Oils are liquids at room temperature. How many types of oils can you find on a grocery shelf? There's corn oil, safflower oil, sesame seed oil, soybean oil, sunflower oil, canola oil, peanut oil, and olive oil. As a general rule, use canola oil for baking and cooking, because it is lowest in saturated fat. Saturated fat will raise your blood cholesterol levels, which increases your risk of heart disease. You can also cook with olive oil because it is a unsaturated oil which tends to lower your blood cholesterol levels.

Salad dressing is used to dress your salad and give it a little spice and pizzazz. Have you ever counted the number of salad dressings on a grocery shelf? Can you graph the number of flavors and the number of fat free, low fat, and regular varieties? Which are your favorites? It might be a good idea to like a few different salad dressings, so you can be flexible when you visit and eat at a friend's house or at a restaurant! What are you in the mood for today? Just remember to like a variety of dressings in moderation! Salad dressings are often high in fat calories.

What's the difference between butter and margarine? Butter is made from animals and contains cholesterol. Margarine is made from vegetable products, e.g., corn or safflower, and does not contain cholesterol. Learn the difference, but realize that both are 100% fat. Does your family use both butter and margarine? Use both sparingly, but go especially easy on the butter because it contains both fat and cholesterol. When your parents buy margarine at the store, do they reach for the sticks of margarine that come in a box or the soft margarine that come in a tub? Soft margarine contains more water and has slightly less fat and calories, so buy the variety that costs the less.

Sweets

Soft drinks and fruit drinks contain plenty of sugar. Drink a variety of beverages by limiting sugary drinks and reaching for water and milk more often. Water is an essential nutrient that you can't live without. Milk helps your bones grow and helps your teeth stay white and strong. Too many sugary drinks will weaken the protective coating on your teeth called enamel.

Sugary cereals are okay to eat in moderation, because cereal is a nutritious food. But on the day that you eat a sugary cereal, try to limit putting jelly, jam, or honey on your bread. Or also avoid drinking sugary soft drinks that day. Eat sweet foods sparingly and not everyday. Sweet foods and drinks contain minimal nutrients, if any. They are often called "empty calories". What's your favorite flavor of jelly or jam? Why is it so easy to like sweet-tasting foods?

Have you ever counted the number of different kinds of candy in a store? Now that's incredible! What's a good rule for including candy in your diet? No, your body doesn't *need* it. But when you *want* to eat some candy, it should be on a day when you haven't eaten other sugary foods and drinks.

Lesson Concept for Grade 2

Important Concepts to Teach about the
Fats, Oils, & Sweets Group

Second Grade Concept — Moderation

Eat Occasionally (Use Sparingly)	<u>Fats and Oils</u> Butter Cream and cream sauce Gravy Lard Margarine Mayonnaise Oil Salad dressing Shortening
Eat Occasionally (Use Sparingly)	<u>Condiments</u> Barbecue sauce Catsup Horseradish Mustard Olives Pickles Salt Soy sauce Taco sauce
Eat Occasionally (Use Sparingly)	<u>Sweets</u> Candy Honey Jellies and Jams Sugar Syrup Soft drinks Fruit drinks

Lesson Concept for Grade 3

Important Concepts to Teach about the Fats, Oils, & Sweets Group

Third Grade Concept — Serving Sizes

Foods in this category supply energy (calories) and flavor, but they are not good sources of nutrients. These foods can be used to enhance your diet, but should not replace foods from the other five food groups. Use these foods occasionally (sparingly). Because Fats, Oils, & Sweets do not provide key nutrients in your diet, there are no recommended serving sizes.

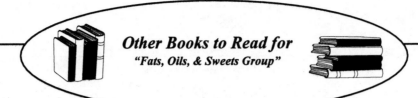

Other Books to Read for
"Fats, Oils, & Sweets Group"

This list contains excellent books to read for learning about the Fats, Oils, & Sweets Group.
Use these books along with the Featured Book when teaching the concepts on the previous pages.

Ahlberg, J., & Ahlberg, A. (1978). Each peach pear plum. New York: Puffin Books.
> A peach, pear, and plum spy on Tom Thumb. Then the story continues with each folktale spying on another. It lists about ten different fairy tales including Cinderella, Robin Hood, The Three Bears, Baby Bunting, Bo-Peep, Jack and Jill and so on.

Balian, L. (1994). The sweet touch. Watertown, WI: Humbug Books.
> Peggy gets a genuine plastic gold ring that brings her a genie. The genie grants Peggy a wish -- everything she touches turns into sweets. Peggy gets a tummy-ache and wants the spell to end. The genie's mother reverses the spell.

Barrett, J. (1986). Pickles have pimples. New York: Macmillan Children's Book Group.
> For example, "Ice cream have cones, birthdays have cakes, sodas have sips, and potatoes have chips."

Barrett, J. (1978). Cloudy with a chance of meatballs. New York: Scholastic Inc.
> As Grandpa is preparing pancakes for his family, a pancake flies across the room which reminds him of a story. He tells his family about a far away land with strange weather that comes three times a day. Whatever falls from the sky is what everyone eats for that day.

Hennessy, B. G. (1992). Jake baked the cake. New York: Scholastic Inc.
> Jake bakes a cake while everyone prepares for the wedding. Everyone at the wedding eats the cake and enjoys it. Jake is proud of his work.

Hennessy, B. G. (1991). The missing tarts. New York: Scholastic Inc.
> The Knave of Hearts stole tarts from the Queen of Hearts. With the help of other nursery rhyme friends, the Queen finds that the Knave of Hearts has given them all away.

Hoban, R. (1981). The great gum drop. New York: Philomel Books.
> Three boys imagine that they are deep sea diving. The oldest boy wants a gum drop, but the middle boy will not share. While they are fighting, the other boy takes all the gumdrops and eats them. They finally make up and have dinner with their parents.

Jaspersohn, W. (1993). Cookies. New York: Macmillan Children's Book Group.
> Cookies are a favorite snack for many people. In this book, you'll discover where cookies are made, what they are made of, and some of the famous cookie companies. (Non-fiction).

Other Books to Read,
Continued

Leedy, L. (1994). The edible pyramid: Good eating every day. New York: Holiday House.
  The Edible Pyramid restaurant opens as the maitre d' explains the food pyramid menu to the
  customers. The maitre d' discusses which foods are included in each group. He also discusses
  how many servings from each group should be eaten everyday.

Lent, B. (1992). Molasses flood. Boston: Houghton Mifflin Co.
  Charley loves molasses! One day the tank of molasses explodes and covers all the streets of
  Boston. His family stocks up on molasses and eats it all the time. Charley finally becomes sick
  of eating molasses.

Mahy, M. (1985). Jam. Boston: Atlantic Monthly.
  A father stays home with the children. The father finds a plum tree, so the family begins making
  jam.

Nixon, J. L. (1986). Beats me, claude. New York: Puffin Books.
  Shirley and Claude are a lonely old couple until Tom comes to stay with them. When Shirley
  tries to make a pie, the U.S. Army comes. When everyone eats the pie, they become sick.

Parish, P. (1979). Amelia bedelia helps out. New York: Avon Books.
  Amelia Bedelia and her niece go to help Miss Emma get ready for a lunch party. Miss Emma
  asks them to weed the garden, feed the chickens, stake her bean plants and other various things.
  Amelia misunderstands her wishes by taking them literally and mixes everything up.

Parish, P. (1987). Teach us, amelia bedelia. New York: Scholastic Inc.
  Amelia Bedelia goes to the school to give the principal a message and ends up teaching for the
  day. She follows the teachers directions in an unusual way. The teacher and the kids both enjoy
  her, especially her taffy apples that she gives as a treat.

Parish, P. (1964). Thank-you, amelia bedelia. New York: HarperCollins Children's Books.
  Amelia Bedelia works as a maid for the Rogers and constantly gets things mixed up. For
  example, she removes spots in Mrs. Roger's dress by cutting them out, strings up the beans,
  separates the eggs, and rolls the jelly for a pastry.

Speed, T. (1994). Hattie baked a wedding cake. New York: The Putnam Publishing Group.
  When Hattie bakes a wedding cake, many things get mixed into the cake like a tuba, socks, and
  a wedding ring. The wedding is almost ruined until Hattie saves the day.

Other Books to Read,
Continued

Spurr, E. (1991). The biggest birthday cake in the world. San Diego: Harcourt Brace & Co.
    The richest man in the world is about to turn forty years old. He asks the chefs to make him
    the world's largest birthday cake. He is very greedy and plans to keep it all to himself, but one
    little boy changes his mind. He then decides to share his cake with everyone.

Stock, C. (1990). Christmas time. New York: Macmillan Children's Book Group.
    It is time for Christmas, so the family goes to look for a tree. They find one and take it home to
    decorate it. In preparation for the arrival of Santa, they also bake cookies, sing songs, and
    make hot cocoa.

Stock, C. (1991). Easter surprise. New York: Macmillan Children's Book Group.
    It is Easter vacation, so the family drives to the cabin for a week. They color Easter eggs, go on
    an Easter egg hunt, and find their Easter baskets.

Walton, M.J. (1983). Tea and whoppers. Milwaukee: Raintree Publishers.
    Karen goes to Gwendolyn's house for a tea party. They tell stories, drink tea, and eat whoppers.

Widman, C. (1992). The lemon drop jar. New York: Macmillan Children's Book Group.
    A little girl visits her Aunt Emma, and they enjoy lemon drop candies together. Aunt Emma
    tells the story about how she got a lemon drop jar when she missed the sun while away at school.

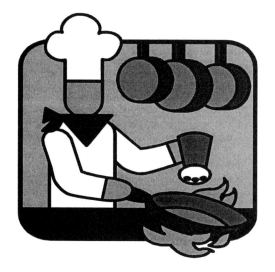

Letter to Food Service Professionals

Our class will be studying a nutrition and health unit called "Building the Food Pyramid". We will learn about the Five Food Groups and practice the important concepts of variety (first graders), moderation (second graders), and serving sizes (third graders). We would like to invite you and/or other members of your staff to our classroom as guest speakers. We would like to learn how you cook and bake foods for us to eat, so we get a variety of different foods as directed by the U.S. Dietary Guidelines for Americans and the Food Guide Pyramid. How do you prepare foods so we get the appropriate serving sizes in moderation? What recipes do you follow for the School Breakfast and Lunch programs? We hope you will be able to talk to us about your work and how you help us to be healthy boys and girls. Our teacher will talk with you soon about your availability during our study of the food pyramid. We hope you might even give us a behind-the-scene tour of the school cafeteria!

Thank you for helping us to learn!

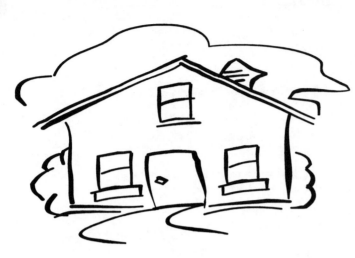

Letter to Parents and Caregivers

Our class will be studying a nutrition and health unit called "Building the Food Pyramid". We will learn about the Five Food Groups and practice the important concepts of variety (first graders), moderation (second graders), and serving sizes (third graders). Anything you can do to help us gather different supplies by _____(date) will be greatly appreciated. Here are some of the items that we need so students will have hands-on, practical learning experiences:

- 1 box of pasta:
    spaghetti
    linguini
    small shell macaroni
    large shell macaroni
    elbow macaroni
    wheel macaroni
    alphabet pasta
    bowtie
    tortellini
    ravioli
    lasagna
    thin noodles
    wide noodles
    angel hair noodles
    ramen noodles
    egg noodles
    tomato pasta
    spinach pasta

- An empty cereal box
- 1 or 2 postage stamps for mailing class letters to request class materials

Thank you kindly!

For the Pleasure of Reading

This booklist can be sent home during Unit 2: Building the Food Pyramid, so that your students and their families can read additional literature about food and nutrition together. You can also place these books in your classroom library during the unit. These books are considered secondary resources for this unit. Each book and its abstract is listed as a primary resource in another unit. Use the index at the back of this book to see how titles are crosslisted with other units. Our goal is to show how each book can be used in multiple ways to teach nutrition and health concepts.

Bread, Cereal, Rice, & Pasta Group
Aliki. (1994). Christmas tree memories. New York: HarperCollins Children's Books.
Carle, E. (1992). Pancakes, pancakes! New York: Scholastic Inc.
Carle, E. (1995). Walter the baker. New York: Simon and Schuster Books for Young Readers.
Czernecki, S., & Rhodes, T. (1992). The sleeping bread. New York: Hyperion Paperbacks.
de Regniers, B. S. (1987). The snow party. New York: Lothrop, Lee and Shepard Books.
dePaola, T. (1978). Pancakes for breakfast. San Diego: Scholastic Inc.
dePaola, T. (1974). Watch out for the chicken feet in your soup. New York: Simon & Schuster
DiSalvo-Ryan, D. (1991). Uncle willie and the soup kitchen. New York: Morrow Junior Books.
Drucker, M. (1992). Grandma's latkes. San Diego: Harcourt Brace & Co.
Forest, H. (1993). The bakers dozen. San Diego: Harcourt Brace & Co.
Garrison, C. (1976). Flim and flam and the big cheese. Scarsdale, NY: Bradbury Press.
Gilman, P. (1990). Grandma and the pirates. New York: Scholastic Inc.
Goldin, B. D. (1988). Just enough is plenty: A hanukkah tale. New York: Puffin Books.
Greeson, J. (1952). The stingy baker. Minneapolis: Carolrhoda Books, Inc.
Hines, A. G. (1988). Daddy makes the best spaghetti. New York: Houghton Mifflin Co.
Ipcar, D. (1976). Hard scrabble harvest. New York: Doubleday & Co., Inc.
Kindersley, D. (1991). My first look at shopping. New York: Random House, Inc.
Kovalski, M. (1990). Pizza for breakfast. New York: Morrow Junior Books.
Lottridge, C. (1990). One watermelon seed. New York: Oxford University Press, Inc.
Manushkin, F. (1992). Latkes and applesauce. New York: Scholastic Inc.
Manushkin, F. (1995). The matzah that papa brought home. New York: Scholastic Inc.
McMillan, B. (1986). Becca backwards, becca frontwards: A book of concept pairs. New York: Lothrop, Lee and Shepard Books.
McMillan, B. (1991). Eating fractions. New York: Scholastic Inc.
Newcome, Z. (1991). Rosie goes shopping. London: Julia MacRae Books.
Nikola-Lisa, W. (1991). 1,2,3 thanksgiving. Morton Grove, IL: Albert Whitman & Company.
Nordgvist, S. (1985). Pancake pie. New York: Morrow Junior Books.
Novak, M. (1990). Mr. floop's lunch. New York: Orchard Books.
Penn, M. (1994). The miracle of the potato latkes. New York: Holiday House Inc.

For the Pleasure of Reading, cont'd

Polacco, P. (1993). The bee tree. New York: Philomel Books.

Polacco, P. (1990). Thunder cake. New York: Scholastic Inc.

Rattigan, J. K. (1993). Dumpling soup. New York: Little, Brown & Co.

Richardson (1991). Stephen's feast. New York: Little, Brown and Company.

Robins, J. (1988). Addie meets max. New York: HarperCollins Children's Books.

Rockwell, H. (1980). My kitchen. New York: Greenwillow Books.

Rose, A. (1973). How does a czar eat potatoes? New York: Lothrop, Lee and Shepard Books.

Rylant, C. (1985). The relatives came. New York: Macmillan Children's Book Group.

Soto, G., & Martinez, E. (1993). Too many tamales. New York: Putnam Publishing Group.

Viorst, J. (1987). Alexander and the terrible, horrible, no good, very bad day. New York: Scholastic.

Walton (1983). Tea and whoppers. Milwaukee: Raintree Publishers.

Watson, W. (1992). Hurray for the fourth of july. New York: Houghton Mifflin Co.

Westcott, N. B. (1988). The lady with the alligator purse. New York: Little, Brown, & Co.

Williams, S. A. (1992). Working cotton. New York: Harcourt Brace & Co.

Wynot, J. (1990). The mother's day sandwich. New York: Orchard Books.

Zimelman, N. (1976). I will tell you of peach stone. New York: Lothrop, Lee, and Shepard Books.

Fruit Group

Altman, L. J. (1993). Amelia's road. New York: Lee & Low Books Inc.

Bang, M. (1984). The grey lady and the strawberry snatcher. New York: Macmillan

Bider, D. (1989). A drop of honey. New York: Simon & Schuster Books for Young Readers.

Bond, R. (1988). Cherry tree. Honesdale, PA: Boyds Hill Press.

DiSalvo-Ryan, D. (1991). Uncle willie and the soup kitchen. New York: Morrow Junior Books.

Florian, D. (1992). A chef. New York: Greenwillow Books.

Garrison, C. (1976). Flim and flam and the big cheese. Scarsdale, NY: Bradbury Press.

Good, E. W. (1994). Fall is here! I love it! Intercourse, PA: Good Books.

Good, E. W. (1990). It's summertime. Intercourse, PA: Good Books.

Hall, Z. (1994). It's pumpkin time! New York: Scholastic Inc.

Hennessy, B. G. (1991). The missing tarts. New York: Scholastic Inc.

Hutchins, P. (1989). Don't forget the bacon. New York: William Morrow & Co., Inc.

Ipcar, D. (1976). Hard scrabble harvest. New York: Doubleday & Co., Inc.

Kimmelman, L. (1989). Frannie's fruits. New York: HarperCollins Children's Books.

Krockover, G., & Krockover, S. (1978). Uncle bill's ice cream shop. New York: Vantage Press.

Levitin (1980). Nobody stole the pie. San Diego: Harcourt Brace & Co.

Lottridge, C. (1990). One watermelon seed. New York: Oxford University Press, Inc.

Manuschkin, F. (1992). Latkes and applesauce. New York: Scholastic Inc.

Merriam, E. (1993). 12 ways to get to 11. New York: Simon and Schuster Books.

Newcome, Z. (1991). Rosie goes shopping. London: Julia MacRae Books.

Nikola-Lisa, W. (1991). 1,2,3 thanksgiving. Morton Grove, IL: Albert Whitman & Company.

Noble, T. H. (1984). Apple tree christmas. New York: Dial Books For Young Readers.

For the Pleasure of Reading, cont'd

Olaleye, I. (1994). Bitter bananas. Honesdale, PA: Boyd's Mill Press.

Polacco, P. (1990). Thunder cake. New York: Scholastic Inc.

Rockwell, A. (1994). Apples and pumpkins. New York: Scholastic Inc.

Rylant, C. (1985). The relatives came. New York: Macmillan Children's Book Group.

Salt, J., & Hawksley, G. (1990). First words and pictures. New York: Larousse Kingfisher Inc.

Saunders, S. (1982). Fish fry. New York: Puffin Books.

Scheffler, U. (1990). The giant apple. Minneapolis: Carolrhoda Books, Inc.

Slawson, M. B. (1994). Apple picking time. New York: Crown Publishers.

Titherington, J. (1990). Pumpkin pumpkin. New York: Scholastic Inc.

Valens, A. (1993). Danilo the fruitman. New York: Dial Books For Young Readers.

Van Woerkom, D. (1975). Becky and the bear. New York: G.P. Putnam's Sons.

Watson, P., & Watson, M. (1994). The market lady and the mango tree. New York: Wm Morrow.

Watson, W. (1992). Hurray for the fourth of july. New York: Houghton Mifflin Co.

Wilder, L. I. (1994). Winter days in the big woods. New York: HarperCollins Children's Books.

Williams, V. B. (1991). Cherries and cherry pits. New York: Scholastic Inc.

Wynot, J. (1990). The mother's day sandwich. New York: Orchard Books.

Zimelman, N. (1976). I will tell you of peach stone. New York: Lothrop, Lee, and Shepard Books.

Vegetable Group

Altman, L. J. (1993). Amelia's road. New York: Lee & Low Books Inc.

Creedle, E. (1934). Down down the mountain. New York: Elscuier/Nelson Books.

DiSalvo-Ryan, D. (1991). Uncle willie and the soup kitchen. New York: Morrow Junior Books.

Drucker, M. (1992). Grandma's latkes. San Diego: Harcourt Brace & Co.

Florian, D. (1992). A chef. New York: Greenwillow Books.

Fowler, A. (1994). Corn-on and off the cob. Chicago: Childrens Press.

Garrison, C. (1976). Flim and flam and the big cheese. Scarsdale, NY: Bradbury Press.

Giovanni, N. (1994). Knoxville, tennessee. New York: Scholastic Inc.

Good, E. W. (1994). Fall is here! I love it! Intercourse, PA: Good Books.

Good, E. W. (1990). It's summertime. Intercourse, PA: Good Books.

Hall, Z. (1994). It's pumpkin time! New York: Scholastic Inc.

Ipcar, D. (1976). Hard scrabble harvest. New York: Doubleday & Co., Inc.

Kimmelman, L. (1989). Frannie's fruits. New York: HarperCollins Children's Books.

Kindersley, D. (1991). My first look at shopping. New York: Random House, Inc.

Krauss, R. (1989). The carrot seed. New York: Scholastic Inc.

Lottridge, C. (1990). One watermelon seed. New York: Oxford University Press, Inc.

Manushkin, F. (1995). The matzah that papa brought home. New York: Scholastic Inc.

McDonald, M. (1994). The potato man. New York: Orchard Books.

McGovern, A. (1986). Stone soup. New York: Scholastic Inc.

Nikola-Lisa, W. (1991). 1,2,3 thanksgiving. Morton Grove, IL: Albert Whitman & Company.

Palmisciano, D. (1989). Garden partners. New York: Antheneum Books for Young Readers.

For the Pleasure of Reading, cont'd

Parish, P. (1964). Thank-you, amelia bedelia. New York: HarperCollins Children's Books.

Penn, M. (1994). The miracle of the potato latkes. New York: Holiday House Inc.

Pochocki, E. (1993). The mushroom man. New York: Simon & Schuster Books.

Rattigan, J. K. (1993). Dumpling soup. New York: Little, Brown & Co.

Rockwell, A. (1994). Apples and pumpkins. New York: Scholastic Inc.

Rose, A. (1973). How does a czar eat potatoes? New York: Lothrop, Lee and Shepard Books.

Salt, J., & Hawksley, G. (1990). First words and pictures. New York: Larousse Kingfisher.

Scheffler, U. (1990). The giant apple. Minneapolis: Carolrhoda Books, Inc.

Shiefman, V. (1994). Sunday potatoes, monday potatoes. New York: Simon & Schuster.

Stock, C. (1990). Thanksgiving treat. New York: Macmillan Children's Book Group.

Titherington, J. (1990). Pumpkin pumpkin. New York: Scholastic Inc.

Watts, B. (1987). Potato. Morristown, NJ: Silver Burdett Press.

Watts, B. (1989). Tomato. Englewood Cliffs, NJ: Silver Burdett Press.

Wilder, L. I. (1994). Winter days in the big woods. New York: HarperCollins Children's Books.

Williams, B. (1978). Jeremy isn't hungry. New York: Dutton Children's Books.

Williams, S. A. (1992). Working cotton. New York: Harcourt Brace & Co.

Milk, Yogurt, & Cheese Group

Brooks, B. (1991). Lemonade parade. Morton Grove, IL: Albert Whitman & Company.

Carle, E. (1992). Pancakes, pancakes! New York: Scholastic Inc.

DiSalvo-Ryan, D. (1991). Uncle willie and the soup kitchen. New York: Morrow Junior Books.

Florian, D. (1992). A chef. New York: Greenwillow Books.

Garrison, C. (1976). Flim and flam and the big cheese. Scarsdale, NY: Bradbury Press.

Giovanni, N. (1994). Knoxville, tennessee. New York: Scholastic Inc.

Good, E. W. (1990). It's summertime. Intercourse, PA: Good Books.

Hest, A. (1994). The midnight eaters. New York: Macmillan Children's Book Group.

Krockover, G., & Krockover, S. (1978). Uncle bill's ice cream shop. New York: Vantage Press.

Kroll, S. (1989). The hokey-pokey man. New York: Holiday House Inc.

McMillan, B. (1986). Becca backwards, becca frontwards: A book of concept pairs. New York.

Novak, M. (1990). Mr. floop's lunch. New York: Orchard Books.

Obligado, L. (1993). The chocolate cow. New York: Simon & Schuster Books for Young Readers.

Polacco, P. (1990). Thunder cake. New York: Scholastic Inc.

Rockwell, H. (1980). My kitchen. New York: Greenwillow Books.

Salt, J., & Hawksley, G. (1990). First words and pictures. New York: Larousse Kingfisher.

Sendak, M. (1970). In the night kitchen. New York: HarperCollins Children's Books.

Van Leeuwen, J. (1974). Too hot for ice cream. New York: Dial Books For Young Readers.

Watson, W. (1992). Hurray for the fourth of july. New York: Houghton Mifflin Co.

Williams, B. (1978). Jeremy isn't hungry. New York: Dutton Children's Books.

Wynot, J. (1990). The mother's day sandwich. New York: Orchard Books.

For the Pleasure of Reading, cont'd

Meat, Poultry, Fish, Dry Beans, Eggs, & Nuts Group

Adams, J. (1991). Going for oysters. Morton Grove, IL: Albert Whitman & Company.

Agnew, S. M. (1970). The giant sandwich. Garden City: Doubleday & Co., Inc.

Baron-Hall, D. (1989). Only at the children's table. Chathem, NJ: Raintree Steck-Vaughn.

Bider, D. (1989). A drop of honey. New York: Simon & Schuster Books for Young Readers.

Carle, E. (1992). Pancakes, pancakes! New York: Scholastic Inc.

Cohen, B. (1987). The carp in the bathtub. Rockville, MD: Kar-Ben Copies, Inc.

DiSalvo-Ryan, D. (1991). Uncle willie and the soup kitchen. New York: Morrow Junior Books.

Drucker, M. (1992). Grandma's latkes. San Diego: Harcourt Brace & Co.

Florian, D. (1992). A chef. New York: Greenwillow Books.

Garrison, C. (1976). Flim and flam and the big cheese. Scarsdale, NY: Bradbury Press.

Goldin, B. D. (1988). Just enough is plenty: A hanukkah tale. New York: Puffin Books.

Howard, E. F. (1991). Aunt flossie's hat (and crab cakes later). New York: Dell Publishers Co, Inc.

Hutchins, P. (1989). Don't forget the bacon. New York: William Morrow & Co., Inc.

Ipcar, D. (1976). Hard scrabble harvest. New York: Doubleday & Co., Inc.

Luenn, N. (1990). Nessa's fish. New York: Scholastic Inc.

McGovern, A. (1986). Stone soup. New York: Scholastic Inc.

McKissack, P.C. (1992). A million fish... more or less. New York: Knopf Books for Young Readers.

Newcome, Z. (1991). Rosie goes shopping. London: Julia MacRae Books.

Nikola-Lisa, W. (1991). 1,2,3 thanksgiving. Morton Grove, IL: Albert Whitman & Company.

Nordgvist, S. (1985). Pancake pie. New York: Morrow Junior Books.

Novak, M. (1990). Mr. floop's lunch. New York: Orchard Books.

Parish, P. (1964). Thank-you, amelia bedelia. New York: HarperCollins Children's Books.

Polacco, P. (1992). Chicken sunday. New York: Scholastic Inc.

Polacco, P. (1988). Rechenka's eggs. New York: Philomel Books.

Polacco, P. (1990). Thunder cake. New York: Scholastic Inc.

Rattigan, J. K. (1993). Dumpling soup. New York: Little, Brown & Co.

Rockwell, H. (1980). My kitchen. New York: Greenwillow Books.

Salt, J., & Hawksley, G. (1990). First words and pictures. New York: Larousse Kingfisher.

Schaefer, J. J. (1994). Miranda's day to dance. New York: Macmillan Children's Book Group.

Soto, G., & Martinez, E. (1993). Too many tamales. New York: Putnam Publishing Group.

Stock, C. (1990). Christmas time. New York: Macmillan Children's Book Group.

Stock, C. (1991). Easter surprise. New York: Macmillan Children's Book Group.

Stock, C. (1990). Thanksgiving treat. New York: Macmillan Children's Book Group.

Watson, W. (1992). Hurray for the fourth of july. New York: Houghton Mifflin Co.

Williams, B. (1978). Jeremy isn't hungry. New York: Dutton Children's Books.

Wynot, J. (1990). The mother's day sandwich. New York: Orchard Books.

Yorinks, A. (1986). Louis the fish. New York: Farrar, Straus, & Giroux.

For the Pleasure of Reading, cont'd

Fats, Oils, & Sweets

Agnew, S. M. (1970). The giant sandwich. Garden City: Doubleday & Co., Inc.

Aliki. (1994). Christmas tree memories. New York: HarperCollins Children's Books.

Bang, M. (1984). The grey lady and the strawberry snatcher. New York: Macmillan.

Bider, D. (1989). A drop of honey. New York: Simon & Schuster Books for Young Readers.

Brown, M. (1951). Skipper john's cook. New York: Charles Scribner's Sons.

Budd, L. (1960). The pie wagon. New York: Lothrop, Lee and Shepard Books.

Carle, E. (1992). Pancakes, pancakes! New York: Scholastic Inc.

Darling, B. (1992). Valerie and the silver pear. New York: Macmillan Children's Book Group.

de Regniers, B. S. (1987). The snow party. New York: Lothrop, Lee and Shepard Books.

Degen, B. (1985). Jamberry. New York: Scholastic Inc.

DiSalvo-Ryan, D. (1991). Uncle willie and the soup kitchen. New York: Morrow Junior Books.

Drucker, M. (1992). Grandma's latkes. San Diego: Harcourt Brace & Co.

Florian, D. (1992). A chef. New York: Greenwillow Books.

Forest, H. (1993). The bakers dozen. San Diego: Harcourt Brace & Co.

Garrison, C. (1976). Flim and flam and the big cheese. Scarsdale, NY: Bradbury Press.

Goldin, B. D. (1993). Cakes and miracles: A purim tale. New York: Puffin Books.

Greenaway, K. (1993). A apple pie. Avenal, NJ: Random House Value Publishing, Inc.

Greeson, J. (1952). The stingy baker. Minneapolis: Carolrhoda Books, Inc.

Hutchins, P. (1989). Don't forget the bacon. New York: William Morrow & Co., Inc.

Ipcar, D. (1976). Hard scrabble harvest. New York: Doubleday & Co., Inc.

Joosse, B. M. (1987). Jam day. New York: HarperCollins Children's Books.

Kindersley, D. (1991). My first look at shopping. New York: Random House, Inc.

Krockover, G., & Krockover, S. (1978). Uncle bill's ice cream shop. New York: Vantage Press.

Lakin, P. (1994). Don't forget. New York: William Morrow & Company Inc.

Levitin (1980). Nobody stole the pie. San Diego: Harcourt Brace & Co.

McDonald, M. (1991). A great pumpkin switch. New York: Orchard Books.

McGrath, B. B. (1994). The m & m counting book. Watertown, MA: Charlesbridge Publishing.

McMillan, B. (1991). Eating fractions. New York: Scholastic Inc.

Nikola-Lisa, W. (1991). 1,2,3 thanksgiving. Morton Grove, IL: Albert Whitman & Company.

Olaleye, I. (1994). Bitter bananas. Honesdale, PA: Boyd's Mill Press.

Polacco, P. (1993). The bee tree. New York: Philomel Books.

Polacco, P. (1990). Thunder cake. New York: Scholastic Inc.

Priceman, M. (1994). How to make an apple pie and see the world. New York: Knopf Books.

Richardson (1991). Stephen's feast. New York: Little, Brown and Company.

Saunders, S. (1982). Fish fry. New York: Puffin Books.

Sendak, M. (1970). In the night kitchen. New York: HarperCollins Children's Books.

Viorst, J. (1987). Alexander and the terrible, horrible, no good, very bad day. New York: Scholastic.

Watson, W. (1992). Hurray for the fourth of july. New York: Houghton Mifflin Co.

Wellington, M. (1992). Mr. cookie baker. New York: Dutton Children's Books.

Wilder, L. I. (1994). Winter days in the big woods. New York: HarperCollins Children's Books.

Wynot, J. (1990). The mother's day sandwich. New York: Orchard Books.

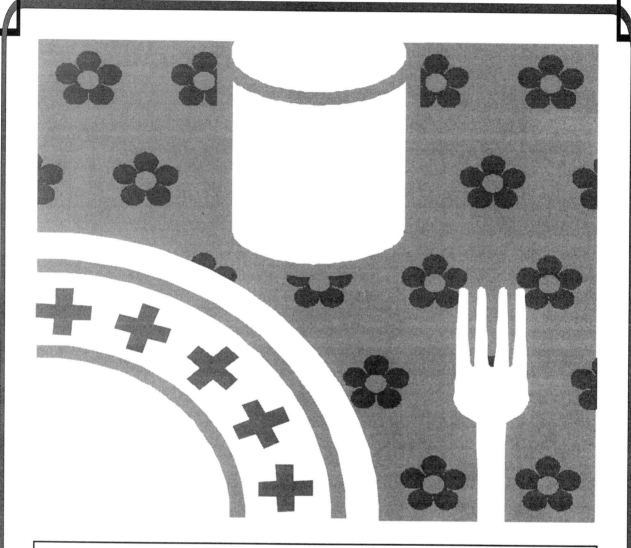

Unit 3:
<u>Let's Make A Meal</u>

**Breakfast, Lunch, and Dinner
Markets, Bakeries, and Vendors
Diners, Restaurants, and Soup Kitchens**

Unit 3: Let's Make a Meal

Instructional activities for Unit 3 have been designed to achieve the *National Health Education Standards*. The performances that students will know and do for this unit are listed below each standard.

⟹ 1. **Students will comprehend concepts related to health promotion and disease prevention.**
   Performance Indicators. As a result of health instruction in Grades K-4, students will
   1. Describe relationships between personal health behaviors and individual well being.
   2. Identify indicators of mental, emotional, social, and physical health during childhood.
   4. Describe how the family influences personal health.
   5. Describe how physical, social, and emotional environments influence personal health.

⟹ 2. **Students will demonstrate the ability to access valid health information and health-promotion products and services.**
   Performance Indicators. As a result of health instruction in Grades K-4, students will
   1. Identify characteristics of valid health information & health-promoting products & services.

⟹ 3. **Students will demonstrate the ability to practice health-enhancing behaviors and reduce health risks.**
   Performance Indicators. As a result of health instruction in Grades K-4, students will
   1. Identify responsible health behaviors.
   2. Identify personal health needs.
   4. Demonstrate strategies to improve or maintain personal health.

⟹ 4. **Students will analyze the influence of culture, media, technology, and other factors on health.**
   Performance Indicators. As a result of health instruction in Grades K-4, students will
   3. Describe ways technology can influence personal health.
   4. Explain how information from school and family influences health.

⟹ 5. **Students will demonstrate the ability to use interpersonal communication skills to enhance health.**
   Performance Indicators. As a result of health instruction in Grades K-4, students will
   3. demonstrate healthy ways to express needs, wants, and feelings.
   4. demonstrate ways to communicate care, consideration, and respect of self & others.
   7. differentiate between negative and positive behaviors used in conflict situations.
   8. demonstrate non-violent strategies to resolve conflicts.

⟹ 6. **Students will demonstrate the ability to use goal setting and decision making skills to enhance health.**
   Performance Indicators. As a result of health instruction in Grades K-4, students will
   1. demonstrate the ability to apply a decision-making process to health issues and problems.

⟹ 7. **Students will demonstrate the ability to advocate for personal, family, & community health.**
   Performance Indicators. As a result of health instruction in Grades K-4, students will
   1. describe a variety of methods to convey accurate health information and ideas.
   2. express information and opinions about health issues.
   3. identify community agencies that advocate for individuals, families, & communitities.
   4. demonstrate the ability to influence and support others in making positive health choices.

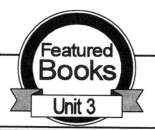

Overall Featured Book for Unit 3

Kelley, T. (1989). Let's eat. New York: Dutton Children's Books.
> Everybody eats. People, animals, and plants all need food. Food comes from many places including the garden, trees, and the sea. There are many different times to eat-breakfast, lunch, dinner, and snacks. Beginning reading level.

Books for Focused Theme: Breakfast, Lunch, and Dinner (Grade 1)

dePaola, T. (1978). Pancakes for breakfast. San Diego: Scholastic Inc.
> A little old lady attempts to have pancakes for breakfast, but she is hindered by a scarcity of supplies and participation of her pets. Beginning reading level.

Hines, A. G. (1991). Jackie's lunch box. New York: William Morrow & Co., Inc.
> While Jackie's sister is at school, Jackie is lonely because she must play by herself. When it is lunchtime, Jackie gets out her lunchbox and eats with her mom. Then Jackie takes a nap until her sister comes home. When her sister gets home, she has a surprise for Jackie. Intermediate reading level.

Sendak, M. (1963). Where the wild things are. New York: HarperCollins Children's Books.
> Max gets sent to his room without dinner. He dreams about a new world of his own where he sails to an island and becomes the king of all the beasts. After all of his fun frolicking with the beasts, he comes home where a hot meal is waiting for him. Intermediate reading level.

Books for Focused Theme: Markets, Bakeries, and Vendors (Grade 2)

Kindersley, D. (1991). My first look at shopping. New York: Random House, Inc.
> There are many things people can buy when they go shopping. At the grocery, there are apples, oranges, peppers, grapes, bananas, corn and lemons. At the bakery, there is cake, croissants, fruit tarts, bread and pastries. There are many other stores to visit too. Low reading level.

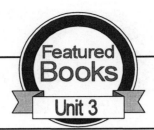

Books for Focused Theme: *Markets, Bakeries, and Vendors, continued*

Carle, E. (1995). <u>Walter the baker</u>. New York: Simon and Schuster Books for Young Readers.
The Duke and Duchess love the sweet rolls prepared by Walter the Baker each morning.
One morning, an accident forces Walter to change his recipe which results in a bad tasting
sweet roll. In order to stay in the kingdom, the Duke orders Walter to create "a roll
through which the rising sun can shine three times, be made from one piece of dough, and
taste good." In his effort to please the Duke and Duchess, and to prevent being banished
from his homeland, Walter creates the pretzel. Advanced reading level.

Kimmelman, L. (1989). <u>Frannie's fruits</u>. New York: HarperCollins Children's Books.
A little girl and her family operate a fruit and vegetable stand near the beach with
the help of their dog, Frannie. She enjoys seeing all the different customers come into
buy different things. Intermediate reading level.

Books for Focused Theme: Diners, Restaurants, & Soup Kitchens (Grade 3)

Loomis, C. (1994). <u>In the diner</u>. New York: Scholastic Inc.
The diner is a busy place. Waiters run around, busboys set the tables, and chefs prepare the
food. Bacon sizzles, coffee brews, bagels toast, burgers broil, and many other things
happen in the busy diner. Low reading level.

Kovalski, M. (1990). <u>Pizza for breakfast</u>. New York: Morrow Junior Books.
Frank and Zeldo own a pizza place. When business gets slow, a strange man appears and
grants them wishes. The pizza place is soon booming and is too much for them to handle.
They decide to try something new so they move to the beach and set up a pizza stand.
Intermediate reading level.

DiSalvo-Ryan, D. (1991). <u>Uncle willie and the soup kitchen</u>. New York: Morrow Junior Books.
A little boy has an Uncle Willie who works at a soup kitchen during the day. The little
boy doesn't understand what a soup kitchen is so Uncle Willie takes him to work. They
prepare and serve a meal to the poor people of the community. Advanced reading level.

Unit 3: Let's Make a Meal
Scope & Sequence of Nutrition Content

Grade 1

Nutrition Content: Dietary Guidelines	*Let's Eat*	*Pancakes for Breakfast*	*Jackie's Lunch Box*	*Where the Wild Things Are*
Eat a variety of foods	X		X	
Balance food with exercise	X	X	X	X
Choose grains, vegetables, and fruits	X	X	X	
Choose low fat and low cholesterol	X	X		
Choose moderate sugars	X	X		
Choose moderate salt and sodium	X			

Nutrition Content: Food Groups	*Let's Eat*	*Pancakes for Breakfast*	*Jackie's Lunch Box*	*Where the Wild Things Are*
Bread, Cereal, Rice, & Pasta Group	X	X	X	
Fruit Group	X		X	
Vegetable Group	X			
Milk, Yogurt, & Cheese Group	X	X	X	
Meat, Poultry, Fish, Dry Beans, Eggs, & Nuts Group	X	X	X	X
Fats, Oils, & Sweets Group	X			X

Unit 3: Let's Make a Meal
Scope & Sequence of Nutrition Content

Grade 2

Nutrition Content: Dietary Guidelines	Let's Eat	My First Look at Shopping	Walter the Baker	Frannie's Fruits
Eat a variety of foods	X			X
Balance food with exercise	X			
Choose grains, vegetables, and fruits	X	X	X	X
Choose low fat and low cholesterol	X			
Choose moderate sugars	X			X
Choose moderate salt and sodium	X			X

Nutrition Content: Food Groups	Let's Eat	My First Look at Shopping	Walter the Baker	Frannie's Fruits
Bread, Cereal, Rice, & Pasta Group	X	X	X	
Fruit Group	X	X		X
Vegetable Group	X	X		X
Milk, Yogurt, & Cheese Group	X		X	
Meat, Poultry, Fish, Dry Beans, Eggs, & Nuts Group	X			
Fats, Oils, & Sweets Group	X	X		

Unit 3: Let's Make a Meal
Scope & Sequence of Nutrition Content

Grade 3

Nutrition Content: Dietary Guidelines	Let's Eat	In the Diner	Pizza for Breakfast	Uncle Willie and the Soup Kitchen
Eat a variety of foods	X			X
Balance food with exercise	X			
Choose grains, vegetables, and fruits	X		X	X
Choose low fat and low cholesterol	X	X		X
Choose moderate sugars	X	X		
Choose moderate salt and sodium	X		X	

Nutrition Content: Food Groups	Let's Eat	In the Diner	Pizza for Breakfast	Uncle Willie and the Soup Kitchen
Bread, Cereal, Rice, & Pasta Group	X	X	X	X
Fruit Group	X		X	X
Vegetable Group	X			X
Milk, Yogurt, & Cheese Group	X	X	X	X
Meat, Poultry, Fish, Dry Beans, Eggs, & Nuts Group	X	X	X	X
Fats, Oils, & Sweets Group	X	X		X

*Overall Featured Book
of Unit 3:
Let's Make a Meal*

Let's Eat!
by True Kelley
Dutton Children's Books, 1989

This lesson addresses the following Dietary Guidelines for Americans:
⇒   *1. Eat a variety of foods.*
⇒   *2. Balance the food you eat with physical activity; maintain or improve your weight.*
⇒   *3. Choose a diet with plenty of grain products, vegetables, and fruits.*
⇒   *4. Choose a diet low in fat, saturated fat, and cholesterol.*
⇒   *5. Choose a diet moderate in sugars.*
⇒   *6. Choose a diet moderate in salt and sodium.*
      7. Choose an alcohol and drug-free lifestyle.

This lesson highlights the following food groups from the Food Guide Pyramid:
⇒   *Bread, Cereal, Rice, & Pasta Group*
⇒   *Fruit Group*
⇒   *Vegetable Group*
⇒   *Milk, Yogurt, & Cheese Group*
⇒   *Meat, Poultry, Fish, Dry Beans, Eggs, & Nuts Group*
⇒   *Fats, Oils, & Sweets*

Food Guide Pyramid
A Guide to Daily Food Choices

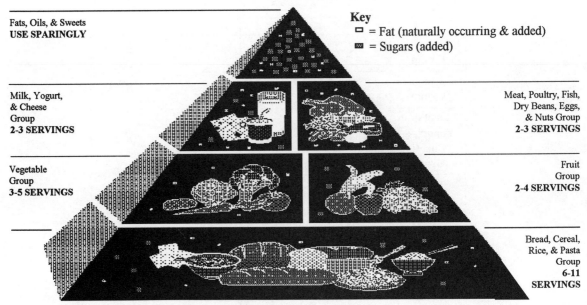

Source: U.S. Department of Agriculture & U.S. Department of Health and Human Services

Lesson Plans for Overall Featured Book

Kelley, T. (1989). <u>Let's eat</u>. New York: Dutton Children's Books.
Everybody eats. People, animals, and plants all need food. Food comes from many places including the garden, trees, and the sea. There are many different times to eat — breakfast, lunch, dinner, and snacks. Beginning reading level.

Pre-Reading Activities for *Let's Eat!*

Write the following words on the chalkboard: What foods do you eat?, Where do you eat?, and With whom do you eat your meals? Brainstorm a list for each category. Compare your class list with the different sections of the book, *Let's Eat!* (MI = I/I)

Create a real or fantasy story about a character who eats a different food in a different place with or without other people. For example, describe how an astronaut would eat breakfast on the moon. (MI = V/L)

Post-Reading Activities for *Let's Eat!*

<u>Questions to develop thinking skills</u> (Bloom's Taxonomy)

1. *Knowledge:*   Name four places where food comes from according to the book.

2. *Comprehension:*   Locate at least five places where you can eat. Discuss one of your more favorite places to eat.

3. *Application:*   Role play an eating situation where you practice good manners. How would you role play an eating situation using bad manners? Report how people felt after watching bad manners.

4. *Analysis:*   Compare your favorite foods for breakfast with your favorite foods for lunch. To what food groups do your favorite foods belong?

5. *Synthesis:*   Plan what you will do today if you are hungry after school and need a snack.

6. *Evaluation:*   Think about how often you eat during a 24-hour period of time. Record the times and places where you usually eat your meals and snacks. Do you notice a pattern from day to day?

Solo Work for *Let's Eat!*

Think about the times of the day when you are hungry, then review the section called Hungry Times in the book. Are you hungry at the same time each day? Does this time vary for you on the weekend? Do you have cravings for a particular food when you wake up in the morning? Do you have any food cravings when you come home from school? What would be your ideal snack after school? Write a couple of sentences for each question. First graders who are just learning to write might dictate their responses into a tape recorder or talk with the teacher or other classroom professional as if they are being interviewed on a talkshow. (MI = I/I, V/L)

Small Group Work for *Let's Eat!*

Compare your answers from above with a friend in your class. Create a comparison chart which shows the similarities and differences you share in the following categories:

Times When Hungry during School
Times When Hungry on the Weekend
Food You Crave in the Morning
Food You Crave After School
Food You Usually Eat After School
Ideal Snack to Eat After School

Did you learn anything new about eating behaviors from your friend? Explain. (MI = I/I, I/S)

Whole Class Work for *Let's Eat!*

Let's explore the social connections we make when we eat with our friends. Place a large piece of butcher paper on a bulletin board, then have your students sign their names on the paper. Help each student tie a long piece of thread to a map pin, then place the pin into the bulletin board next to the student's name. Grab the free end of the string and ask each student who they ate lunch with yesterday. Use another pin to attach the end of the string to the board at another person's name. Use a different colored thread over three days to see the variety of social connections each person makes during lunch time. Discuss how these interactions add a pleasurable element to eating. Also talk about how your social interactions might change from setting to setting. For example, do you have more conversation or less conversation when you are on a picnic at the park? Eating at a restaurant? Eating in the car? And eating at home? Discuss how the types of food that you eat will change from setting to setting. For example, would you eat lobster at the movies? Would you eat ice cream in a canoe? Choose a logical food to eat in a logical place and choose a silly food to eat in an unusual place. Create a short skit with three or four of your classmates, demonstrating either your logical or silly example. Use at least one prop to demonstrate your ideas. (MI = V/S, V/L, I/I, I/S)

Across the Curriculum for *Let's Eat!*

Social Studies

Eating is a fun activity, because we often eat with family and friends. Select two different holidays that your family celebrates. Make a list of foods typical for those holidays. What family traditions help to determine these eating behaviors? (MI = V/L, I/I)

Mathematics

For one day, keep a chart of the foods and beverages you consume and at what time you consume them. Look at the time intervals between your meals, drinks, and snacks. Do you eat small frequent meals throughout the day or fewer, larger meals? What is the average number of times you eat in a day? Calculate how many times you would eat over the course of one week. (MI = L/M, I/I)

Science

For most individuals, a carbohydrate-rich food will take 2 to 3 hours to digest. Protein-rich foods will take approximately 3 to 5 hours to digest, and fat-rich foods will take 6 to 8 hours to digest. Some individuals metabolize food faster than others so they will need to eat more frequent meals. What makes your stomach growl? Is it an accurate measure of hunger for you? (MI = L/M, V/L)

Language Arts

Create an "I Remember When Story" about food. Use the Food Tricks section of the book for inspiration. (MI = V/L)

Physical Education

Let's play! Eating and exercise should go hand-in-hand. Try to balance the food you eat with physical activity. You eat every day, so you should be active every day. Choose an activity that is fun to do with one other person. What activity do you like that requires more than two people? And what activity do you like to do by yourself? Plan lots of fun activities to do. A physically active lifestyle keeps you healthy. Do something now for ten minutes in your classroom or go outside! (MI = I/I, B/K)

Art

Collect a photo from home which shows you eating with friends or family members. Tape the photo to a larger piece of cardboard. Make a dried pasta or cereal border around the photo. Hang to dry. Don't forget to write a caption for your picture! (MI = B/K, V/S, V/L)

Music

Sing the song called "I Wonder if I'm Growing" by Raffi (See the list of Teaching Resources in the back of the book). Role play or pantomime some motions to go with the song.

Across the Curriculum

Focused Theme:
Breakfast, Lunch, and Dinner

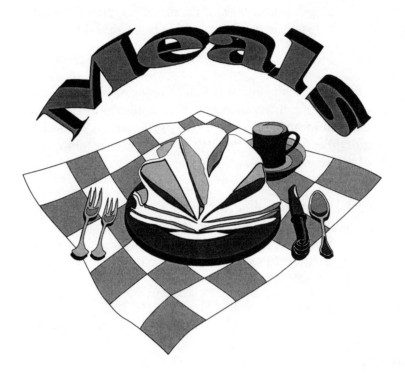

Overview of Breakfast, Lunch, and Dinner:

This focused theme emphasizes our eating behavior during the three major meals of our day, including snacks. Eating behavior is designated by *what* we eat, *when* we eat, *where* we eat, and *with whom* we eat. This section will highlight when we eat. For example, most people eat a morning meal, an afternoon meal, and an evening meal. Some people also eat one or two nutritious snacks during their active day. The feature books in this section also address what kinds of foods and with whom we eat our meals.

Featured Book #1 of the Focused Theme: Breakfast, Lunch, and Dinner	*Pancakes for Breakfast* **by Tomie dePaola Scholastic Inc., 1978**

This lesson addresses the following Dietary Guidelines for Americans:
1. Eat a variety of foods.
⇒ *2. Balance the food you eat with physical activity; maintain or improve your weight.*
⇒ *3. Choose a diet with plenty of grain products, vegetables, and fruits.*
⇒ **4. Choose a diet low in fat, saturated fat, and cholesterol.**
⇒ *5. Choose a diet moderate in sugars.*
6. Choose a diet moderate in salt and sodium.
7. Choose an alcohol and drug-free lifestyle.

This lesson highlights the following food groups from the Food Guide Pyramid:
⇒ *Bread, Cereal, Rice, & Pasta Group*
Fruit Group
Vegetable Group
⇒ *Milk, Yogurt, & Cheese Group*
⇒ *Meat, Poultry, Fish, Dry Beans, Eggs, & Nuts Group*

Food Guide Pyramid
A Guide to Daily Food Choices

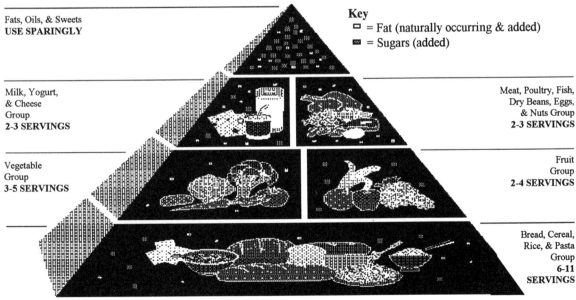

Source: U.S. Department of Agriculture & U.S. Department of Health and Human Services

Lesson Plans for Featured Book 1

dePaola, T. (1978). <u>Pancakes</u> for <u>breakfast</u>. San Diego: Scholastic Inc.
A little old lady attempts to have pancakes for breakfast, but she is hindered by a
scarcity of supplies and participation of her pets. Beginning reading level.

Pre-Reading Activities for *Pancakes for Breakfast*

How many of you ate breakfast today? How many of you ate breakfast yesterday? How many of you plan
to eat breakfast tomorrow? Do you tend to eat breakfast by yourself or with other people? Why?
(MI = I/I, V/L)

What kinds of pancakes do you like? Do they like blueberry pancakes, buttermilk pancakes, buckwheat
pancakes, and potato pancakes (latkes)? Have you ever eaten at a pancake restaurant? Describe your
experience so we feel like we are smelling, seeing, tasting, and touching the food at the restaurant. What
sounds would we hear in the restaurant while eating our pancake meal? (MI = I/I, V/L)

Post-Reading Activities for *Pancakes for Breakfast*

<u>Questions to develop thinking skills</u> (Bloom's Taxonomy)

1. Knowledge:	Name all the ingredients that the woman needed for making pancakes for breakfast.
2. Comprehension:	Explain how this woman's method of making pancakes is different from the method used today.
3. Application:	Report the problem in this story. Then put in order the events that led to the solution of the problem.
4. Analysis:	Observe the number of ingredients for making pancakes in the story. How many food groups are represented? Categorize the different ingredients into the food pyramid.
5. Synthesis:	Create a new routine for the woman so she does not have the same problem the next time she makes pancakes. Can you help the woman get the same amount of physical activity?
6. Evaluation:	Judge the woman's behavior after her pets ruin the pancake for her.

Solo Work for *Pancakes for Breakfast*

Bring a pancake recipe to class from a cookbook or the back of a pancake mix box. Compare the ingredients list from your recipe with the pancake recipe found in the book. Copy the two lists and count the number of steps in each of the pancake recipes. (MI = V/S, L/M)

Small Group Work for *Pancakes for Breakfast*

Within your small group of two to four people, select one of your recipes to be used at a School Pancake Day. Next, take a group vote on your favorite syrup or topping for pancakes. Draw and label the steps required for making the syrup or topping. Also investigate then write the cost of the syrup or topping on an index card then post it near the topping on the School Pancake Day. (MI = I/S, L/M, V/S)

Whole Class Work for *Pancakes for Breakfast*

Collect the selected recipes from each of the small groups and photocopy a complete list to distribute to parents. Attach the recipes to a Parent Letter and ask them if they would be willing to make a pancake recipe at home to be donated to the class. Invite these parents or caregivers to class to assist with a small group of students on School Pancake Day. Also ask them to bring electric skillets to class, if available. You can also ask for help from the food service professionals in your school.

On the School Pancake Day, students can assist with the distribution of plastic-coated paper plates, napkins, and utensils while the electric skillets are heating up. Students can also place the different syrups and toppings on a central table with the index cards with prices displayed next to each. When the electric skillets are coated with adequate oil and are hot, each student will scoop pancake batter from the batter bowl into the skillet for one pancake. Grown-ups will supervise the making of the pancakes and will turn the pancakes in the skillet when they are ready, placing them in a covered casserole dish until all the pancakes are made. After a student has made one pancake, he or she will rotate to another food station to make a different pancake to eat. When all the pancakes are made, students will choose two different pancakes to eat. Second helpings may be available after all students and grown ups have been served. Everyone assists with clean up. Discuss whether the clean up takes less time or more time than the preparation. Ask the grown-ups who made the pancake batter whether they think there is much time difference in making a pancake batter from scratch and making a pancake batter from a box. Do you think there is a difference in taste between pancakes made from scratch and pancakes made from a box? (MI = B/K, I/I, V/L)

Across the Curriculum for *Pancakes for Breakfast*

Social Studies

Compare the history of different breakfast foods that are prepared on a hot grill, e.g., pancakes, French toast, crepes, waffles, and others. For example, crepes originated from France. Did French toast also originate in France? (MI = V/L)

Mathematics

Syrups and toppings for pancakes can be very expensive. Compare the cost of pure maple syrup and artificial syrup which is made with smaller amounts of maple syrup or corn syrup. (MI = L/M)

Science

Did you ever skip breakfast? Just leave your house and not eat anything for breakfast? Or have you ever been late for school and have no time for breakfast? Not a good idea! The human body needs a constant supply of energy to help it run smoothly. If you were a car and you did not have fuel, then you would stop running. The same is true of your body. No fuel, no go. Breakfast is the first meal of day and should supply at least one third of the food you need for that day. Food scientists called dietitians think that it is the most important meal of the day. Read about the role of breakfast in helping you to think, compute, and maintain a good mood. Invite a dietitian to your class to speak about breakfast. (MI = V/L)

Language Arts

Write ten different sentences that describe what you do and how you feel when you wake up in the morning. Where does your breakfast fit into your routine? Do you wash your hands? Brush your teeth? Place each of your ideas on an index card, so you can create a sequence story to share with others. (MI = I/I, V/L, I/S)

Physical Education

The lady in the story is a very fit person! Discuss all the ways that she demonstrated physical fitness in order to make her breakfast. Our lifestyles today are not quite as active. Organize a class fitness club so that you can do an aerobic activity after school or during physical education class. Keep track of the number of minutes that you go walking, running, bicycling, swimming, or other activities during club time. If students exercise at home after school, parents can verify the type and amount of exercise with a signature. To obtain the most aerobic benefits, try to exercise at least three times a week for twenty minutes of continuous activity. (MI = I/S, L/M)

Art

Make a class portfolio showing the number of steps your class went through to prepare then participate in the School Pancake Day. Take photos and draw pictures for a visual memory of the event. Write captions under each picture. You can also use computer software to help stylize your portfolio. (MI = V/S, V/L, B/K)

Music

Modify and substitute the words "pancake cook" in "The Muffin Man" song. Sing the song during the School Pancake Day. Here's the song: "Oh, do you know the pancake cook? The pancake cook? The pancake cook? Oh, do you know the pancake cook, who helps in our great school?" (MI = M/R)

*Featured Book #2
of the Focused Theme:
Breakfast, Lunch, and
Dinner*

Jackie's Lunch Box
by Anna Grossnickle Hines
William Morrow & Co., Inc., 1991

This lesson addresses the following Dietary Guidelines for Americans:

⇒ *1. Eat a variety of foods.*
⇒ *2. Balance the food you eat with physical activity; maintain or improve your weight.*
⇒ *3. Choose a diet with plenty of grain products, vegetables, and fruits.*
   4. Choose a diet low in fat, saturated fat, and cholesterol.
   5. Choose a diet moderate in sugars.
   6. Choose a diet moderate in salt and sodium.
   7. Choose an alcohol and drug-free lifestyle.

This lesson highlights the following food groups from the Food Guide Pyramid:

⇒ *Bread, Cereal, Rice, & Pasta Group*
⇒ *Fruit Group*
   Vegetable Group
⇒ *Milk, Yogurt, & Cheese Group*
⇒ *Meat, Poultry, Fish, Dry Beans, Eggs, & Nuts Group*

Food Guide Pyramid
A Guide to Daily Food Choices

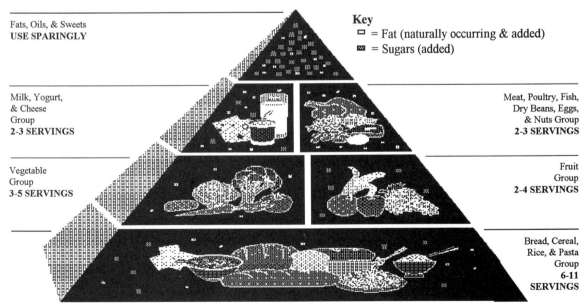

Source: U.S. Department of Agriculture & U.S. Department of Health and Human Services

Lesson Plans for Featured Book 2

Hines, A. G. (1991). <u>Jackie's</u> <u>lunch</u> <u>box</u>. New York: William Morrow & Co., Inc.
While Jackie's sister is at school, Jackie is lonely because she must play by herself. When
it is lunchtime, Jackie gets out her lunchbox and eats with her mom. Then Jackie takes
a nap until her sister comes home. When her sister gets home, she has a surprise for Jackie.
Intermediate reading level.

Pre-Reading Activities for *Jackie's Lunch Box*

It takes time to pack a lunch with nutritious foods! Interview your parent or caregiver who packs your
lunch to go to school or to a sporting event after school. Discuss ways to assist with the process. How
much time can you save if you work together? What foods are just perfect for decreasing the time to make
a lunch in the morning or the night before? Invite a parent or caregiver to class who still packs lunches for
a large family. Make a list of questions you plan to ask. What foods are good for lunch? Where do you
usually keep the lunch boxes (or lunch bags) in your house? When do you pack the lunches? With whom
do you pack the lunches? Why do you pack lunches from home instead of using the School Lunch
program at school? (MI = V/L)

Post-Reading Activities for *Jackie's Lunch Box*

Questions to develop thinking skills (Bloom's Taxonomy)

1. *Knowledge:*   Repeat the sequence of activities that Jackie does while her sister is at school.

2. *Comprehension:*   Explain how Jackie felt about her sister Carla. Use examples from the story.

3. *Application:*   Role play how Jackie's mother would pack two lunch boxes in the morning.

4. *Analysis:*   Examine the items Jackie found in the kitchen. What food groups did she find?
   Which food groups did she not find?

5. *Synthesis:*   Imagine the things that Jackie says to Midgie and Fudge during the day when they
   play school, read a story together, and wait on a blanket in the front yard for
   Carla.

6. *Evaluation:*   Recommend a daily routine for Jackie when it is too cold to play outside. Be sure
   the routine continues to give Jackie exercise.

Solo Work for *Jackie's Lunch Box*

Look at magazines to find pictures of food that you like to eat for lunch. Cut out the pictures and paste them to a paper plate. Try to select a food from each food group. Remember that a sandwich is a combination food, which crosses into more than one food group. Jackie's peanut butter sandwich includes a serving from the Bread, Cereal, Rice, & Pasta Group and a serving from the Meat, Poultry, Fish, Dry Beans, Eggs, & Nuts Group. Jackie's lunch also included a banana, two cookies, and some milk. Decide what food group is missing from Jackie's lunch. Can you think of some examples that Jackie could eat? She doesn't really need to eat vegetables during her lunch as long as she gets some vegetables during her other meals or snacks that day. What food group is missing from your paper plate? See if you can find a picture of a food from that food group. Paste it to the back of your plate as a reminder for eating later in the day. (MI = B/K, V/S)

Small Group Work for *Jackie's Lunch Box*

Sandwiches originated in the early 1700's when John Montagu, Britain's fourth Earl of Sandwich, combined different kinds of food between two slices of bread. Sandwiches have been created in other cultures too. In the Middle East, people make pita or pocket bread sandwiches. In Mexico, people make tacos or burritos. In Italy, people make calizones. And in China, people make egg rolls. Within your small groups of three to four students, brainstorm a list of your favorite sandwiches. According to a recent survey by Market Research Institute for IronKids Bread, the top five sandwiches in the last few years were peanut butter and jelly; ham and cheese; bologna and cheese; turkey; and tuna fish. After you take a vote among your small group members, take a class vote to see if you agree with these national findings. (MI = I/S, L/M)

Whole Class Work for *Jackie's Lunch Box*

Plan a Sandwich Celebration for your class in which a variety of sandwiches from different food groups are made at home then eaten during lunch at school. Have you ever eaten different fruit and vegetable sandwiches? Who will volunteer to make a tomato sandwich? A cucumber sandwich? An avocado sandwich? Have you ever eaten different protein sandwiches besides peanut butter? Who will volunteer to make an egg salad sandwich? Who will volunteer to make a cheese sandwich? Who will volunteer to make a roast beef sandwich? Of course, some of you will want to make a few of your favorite sandwiches too.

Each student is to bring a whole sandwich to class that is uncut. Sort the sandwiches onto one large cutting board for energy and maintenance sandwiches (representing the Bread Group, Fruit Group, and Vegetable Group from Unit 2) and onto one large cutting board for body-building sandwiches (representing the Bread Group, the Milk, Yogurt, & Cheese Group, and the Meat, Poultry, Fish, Dry Beans, Eggs, & Nuts Group). Take turns cutting a sandwich into four equal pieces, then arranging the quarters onto serving trays or plates. Perhaps you can cut a variety of square and triangle sandwiches.

At lunch time, everyone eats together in the classroom or outdoors if the weather is nice. Students will eat the other food in their lunch that they brought to school, but they will share their sandwiches so everyone can taste a variety of different kinds. During lunch, talk about how you feel when you eat with other people. How do you like tasting a variety of different sandwiches? Try to use some of the following polite statements during lunch: "This sandwich is delicious." "This sandwich tastes good." "This sandwich is not my favorite kind, but I'll eat it for a change." (MI = B/K, L/M, I/S, V/L)

Across the Curriculum for *Jackie's Lunch Box*

Social Studies

Have you ever forgotten your lunch at home when you're in a hurry? What happened? Did you still get to eat lunch? How? Talk about what construction workers might do when they forget their lunch. What do you suppose office workers do? What type of lunch boxes or bags do your parents or caregivers take to work? (MI = V/L)

Mathematics

Bread is packaged in many different types of wrappers, bags, and sacks. Compare the different weight and prices of five different loaves of bread. Don't be fooled by the size of the loaf! Which loaf is the best deal? (MI = L/M)

Science

Why should you use insulated lunch bags for your lunch? Estimate the length of time between when your lunch is made and when your lunch is eaten. Why are paper bags and plastic bags not as good for storing your lunch if a refrigerator is not available? The same holds true if you bring your food home from the grocery store in paper or plastic bags. That's why some frozen foods are double bagged for you, often upon your request if you know you won't be driving right home. (MI = L/M, V/L)

Language Arts

Tell a story about your favorite place to eat lunch. Use a tape recorder to record your story. Ask a classmate to repeat your story from memory. Play back your tape recorded message to compare your version of the story with your classmate's story. Switch roles and don't forget to tell why you like to eat lunch at your favorite place. (MI = V/L, I/S)

Physical Education

Show different stunts or skills you can practice while waiting at the bus stop like Carla does in the story. Can you march in place or shuffle your feet? How do these stunts or skills change if there is more than one person waiting with you? Can you jump over a ball rolled toward you? What non-locomotor activity can you do while standing in the food line in the school lunch room? Can you stand on one leg without falling over? Can you stand on tiptoe and stretch for the ceiling? (MI = B/K)

Art

Talk about the concept of perspective in art. Look at the drawing of Jackie's lunch box on the dedication page of the book. Notice how the artist gave us a view of the lunch box so it looks real. How did she do that? See if you can draw a lunch box. Perhaps you can use watercolor paints and colored pencils like the illustrator did. (MI = V/L, V/S)

Music

Learn the Raffi song called "Peanut Butter Sandwich" (See Teaching Resources at the end of the book). It might be fun to sing the song during your Sandwich Celebration. Maybe you'd like to create other songs about bologna sandwiches, bean sprout sandwiches, and pastrami sandwiches. Have some silly fun! (MI = M/R)

Across the Curriculum

<table>
</table>

Featured Book #3 of the Focused Theme: *Breakfast, Lunch, and Dinner*	*Where the Wild Things Are* by Maurice Sendak HarperCollins Children's Books, 1963

This lesson addresses the following Dietary Guidelines for Americans:

1. Eat a variety of foods.
⇒ 2. *Balance the food you eat with physical activity; maintain or improve your weight.*
3. Choose a diet with plenty of grain products, vegetables, and fruits.
4. Choose a diet low in fat, saturated fat, and cholesterol.
5. Choose a diet moderate in sugars.
6. Choose a diet moderate in salt and sodium.
7. Choose an alcohol and drug-free lifestyle.

This lesson highlights the following food groups from the Food Guide Pyramid:

Bread, Cereal, Rice, & Pasta Group
Fruit Group
Vegetable Group
⇒ *Milk, Yogurt, & Cheese Group*
⇒ *Meat, Poultry, Fish, Dry Beans, Eggs, & Nuts Group*

Food Guide Pyramid
A Guide to Daily Food Choices

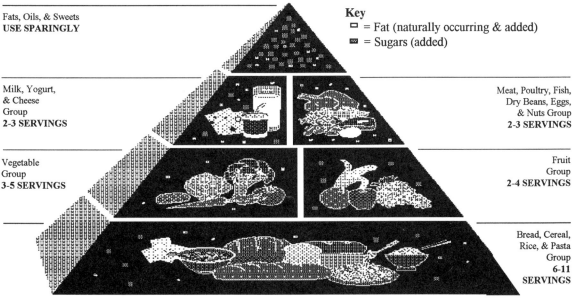

Source: U.S. Department of Agriculture & U.S. Department of Health and Human Services

Lesson Plans for Featured Book 3

Sendak, M. (1963). <u>Where the wild things are</u>. New York: HarperCollins Children's Books.
Max gets sent to his room without dinner. He dreams about a new world of his own where
he sails to an island and becomes the king of all the beasts. After all of his fun frolicking with
the beasts, he comes home where a hot meal is waiting for him. Intermediate reading level.

Pre-Reading Activities for *Where the Wild Things Are*

Discuss an exotic place or an adventuresome trip that you have visited or imagined. How did you get
there? What did you eat? When did you eat it? (MI = V/L)

Post-Reading Activities for *Where the Wild Things Are*

Questions to develop thinking skills (Bloom's Taxonomy)

1. Knowledge: Tell why Max was sent to his room.

2. Comprehension: Discuss what name you give your evening meal. Do you eat dinner or
                          supper?

3. Application: Illustrate a ten-step timeline showing Max's feelings over the course of
                          his adventure. Use faces to depict his changing emotions.

4. Analysis: Which wild thing would you be willing to meet at a restaurant for dinner?
                          Why? Compare your choice with another person's choice.

5. Synthesis: Narrate some words to go with the pages of the book which have pictures
                          only.

6. Evaluation: Consider the negative effects on Max if he did not receive his dinner at all
                          in the story. How might Max's emotions or behaviors change if he was
                          really hungry after his adventure?

Solo Work for *Where the Wild Things Are*

What makes you feel secure and happy in your family? Hugs? Food when you are hungry? A house to live in? A bed to sleep in? A stuffed animal or pet? Explain how you feel when one of these things is taken away from you. Make a thank you card for a parent or sibling or other caregiver to show your appreciation and love for them. (MI = V/L, V/S)

Small Group Work for *Where the Wild Things Are*

Sometimes our parents and caregivers say "Eat your dinner or you will not get any desert". Dinner is an important meal because it usually contains foods from all of the different food groups. By eating dinner, you will often get all the important nutrients your body needs to stay healthy. There are many healthful deserts to have after dinner or sometimes even with your dinner. Within your small group of three or four students, decide whether the following deserts are "okay to eat during a meal" or "better to eat after the meal":

Fresh sliced strawberries in a bowl
Chocolate cake
Ice cream
Fresh sliced peaches in a bowl
Pudding
Graham crackers
Cookies and milk
Sliced cantaloupe

After you have decided when to eat these deserts in relationship to dinner, review the list again and decide where the food belongs on the food pyramid. Just like dinner foods, some deserts contain more than one food group. For example, banana pudding with vanilla wafers would fit into two food groups: Milk, Yogurt, & Cheese Group and Bread, Cereal, Rice, & Pasta Group. (MI = I/S, V/L)

Whole Class Work for *Where the Wild Things Are*

In the story, Max came home from his wild adventure to find his supper waiting for him. He has a smile on his face and he looks content, knowing that he is in the security of his home and in the warmth of his mother's love. When we meet unexpected events in our life, it's always good to know that we can feel safe, protected, and cared for. How many of you felt uneasy or even scared when Max first met the wild things? Did your fears stay the same through the whole story? How do you feel after you read the story a second time? A third time? A fourth time? Do your fears stay the same?

Learning to accept something that is unfamiliar to us takes time. In nutrition, experts have found that children can have a reluctance or fear to try new foods. Food preferences develop slowly, and "often children must have ten exposures to a food before they're willing to accept it" (Birch et al, 1995). Unfortunately, adults may give up offering a food to a child after a few times. Have you ever gone to a grocery store on a weekend when there are people serving small bites of new food products? Were you willing to try the new foods? Most people will try something once, especially if they are hungry! Have you ever gone to a large Taste Festival in your city? At Taste Festivals, many restaurants sell smaller portions of their favorite foods. A favorite food for one person may not be a favorite food for another person. That's why there are so many different (variety) foods at Taste Festivals!

Invite a dietitian to come to your class to "taste-test" some new food products. You may also volunteer to taste test any foods that older students make in home economics class in your school district. The lesson to be learned is to try new foods with a sense of adventure. Max sure demonstrated a sense of adventure when he traveled to "where the wild things are"!! (MI = V/L, B/K)

Across the Curriculum for *Where the Wild Things Are*

Social Studies

When Max went on his travels, he did not take any food or water with him. According to the story, he "sailed back over a year and in and out of weeks and through a day." Is it possible for Max to go that long without food and water? How did people eat long ago when they had to travel long distances on foot, by horse, or by covered wagon? How did they carry or find their food? (MI = V/L)

Mathematics

Make a chart that shows how many new foods you tried during a recent Taste Festival. Create your own rating system so that you will know your favorite food at the end of the event. Have another serving of your favorite food before you go home. But why don't you try your least favorite food one more time too? Your favorite food can be your reward after that! (MI = B/K, L/M)

Science

If you travel a long distance, you use coolers to keep your food cool. There are even insulated heaters for keeping your food warm. Experiment with different types of ice to use in your cooler. What type of ice will help keep your food cold the longest? Crushed ice, small cubes, or large cubes? Why would the large cubes last the longer? What happens to the ice when you keep opening the cooler (or the refrigerator at home)? (MI = V/L, L/M)

Language Arts

Make flash cards for different feelings. On one side of the card, draw a face showing a feeling or an expression. Some suggested words include surprise, afraid, angry, excited, upset, frustrated, and sad. Be sure to include some of the words that describe Max's changing emotions in the story. On the other side of the card, write a word to describe the feeling. Each day have a student select a card to role play in front of class. Once the class guesses the feeling that is role played, say the word aloud several times and practice spelling the word. In your class writing journal, write a sentence using the new vocabulary word. (MI = V/L, B/K, I/S)

Physical Education

Create your own "wild thing" aerobic dance to music. Use hopping, marching, jogging, jumping, skipping, kicking, and clapping. (MI = B/K, M/R)

Art

Draw a mural or frieze of wild things eating new and different foods with Max. Use ink to add lines and details to your drawing like the illustrator, Maurice Sendak, did. Why do the illustrations get larger then smaller in the book? (MI = V/S, V/L)

Music

Add percussion accompaniment to the music you select for your "wild thing" aerobic dance. While some students are doing the aerobic dance, other students can add rhythm and sound. (MI = M/R)

Across the Curriculum

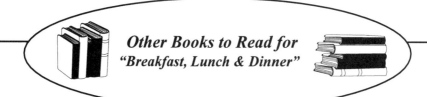

***Other Books to Read for
"Breakfast, Lunch & Dinner"***

This list contains excellent books to read for learning about Breakfast, Lunch, & Dinner. Use these books along with the Featured Books when teaching the lessons on the previous pages.

Agnew, S. M. (1970). <u>The giant sandwich</u>. Garden City: Doubleday & Co., Inc.
> Mr. Magoffin is hungry so he decides to make a sandwich. He tastes each item to make sure he wants it on his sandwich. When his sandwich is made, he is no longer hungry.

Aliki. (1994). <u>Christmas tree memories</u>. New York: HarperCollins Children's Books.
> A family shares memories about each Christmas ornament on their tree made of dough, walnuts, and corn husks. Many memories center around family gatherings at mealtime.

Breinburg, P. (1974). <u>Doctor shawn</u>. New York: Thomas Y. Crowell Company.
> Mom went shopping, so Shawn and his sisters decide to play doctor. Shawn is the doctor and he bandages all the patients all day long. Then mother comes home and tells them to close the hospital, because it is time for lunch.

Caines, J. (1988). <u>I need a lunchbox</u>. New York: Scholastic Inc.
> A little boy wants a lunchbox very badly. He feels sad because he can't have one until he starts school like his sister. In the end, his father surprises him with a lunchbox.

Carle, E. (1992). <u>Pancakes, pancakes</u>! New York: Scholastic Inc.
> A rooster crows to wake Jack. Jack decides he wants pancakes for breakfast. Jack has to go cut the wheat and grind it. Then he gets an egg from a chicken and some milk from a cow. Next he gets firewood and finally it is time to make pancakes.

Carle, E. (1993). <u>Today is monday</u>. New York: Scholastic Inc.
> Today is Monday and it is string bean day. Tuesday is spaghetti day and Wednesday is ZOOOOP. Thursday is roast beef and Friday is fresh fish. It is time for all the hungry children to eat up!

Cohen, B. (1988). <u>Don't eat too much turkey</u>. New York: Dell Publishing Co., Inc.
> It is almost Thanksgiving. The first grade builds a class turkey together, then takes turns pretending to be the turkey. Preparations are also made for the children's turkey dinner at home.

Dalton, A. (1992). <u>This is the way</u>. New York: Scholastic Inc.
> A family goes through the routine of their day in the rhythm of the tune "here we go round the mulberry bush".

Other Books to Read,
Continued

Garrison, C. (1976). <u>Flim and flam and the big cheese</u>. Scarsdale, NY: Bradbury Press.
    Two brothers, one fat and one thin, live together. Flam eats all the food and leaves
    nothing for Flim. So Flim decides to trick Flam into drinking the pond by placing a
    piece of cheese in the middle of it. Flam drinks the whole pond not realizing the cheese was
    the reflection of the moon. Since Flam cannot move, Flim is able to eat a very satisfying meal.

Hennessy, B. G. (1992). <u>School days</u>. New York: Scholastic Inc.
    Children do many things in school. There is circle time, letter and rhyming games,
    telling time, fire drill, reading, writing, recess, lunchtime, storytime and riding the bus home.

Hines, A. G. (1988). <u>Daddy makes the best spaghetti</u>. New York: Houghton Mifflin Co.
    A little boy and his dad go to the grocery store to get food for dinner. They decide to make
    spaghetti, so they buy noodles and sauce. When they get home, they make dinner with his mom.
    After they eat and do the dishes, his dad carries him to bed.

Hines, A. G. (1991). <u>The greatest picnic in the world</u>. New York: Clarion Books.
    It is picnic time with turkey sandwiches, mustard, cheese, pickles, crackers, cheese
    nips, chocolate chips, celery sticks, apples, grapes and hard-boiled eggs. It begins to rain, so
    everything is packed back into the car. The picnic continues inside.

Howard, J. R. (1992). <u>When i'm hungry</u>. New York: Dutton Children's Books.
    When I am hungry I like to eat. The little boy in this book uses his imagination at mealtime.
    He wonders what it would be like to eat underwater, to eat in the mud, to dive for his food,
    and to store food in his cheeks.

Kindersley, D. (1991). <u>My first look at time</u>. New York: Random House, Inc.
    Important times of a child's day are highlighted from nutrition to hygiene.

Leedy, L. (1994). <u>The edible pyramid: Good eating every day</u>. New York: Holiday House.
    The Edible Pyramid restaurant opens as the maitre d' explains the food pyramid menu to
    the customers. The maitre d' discusses which foods are included in each group. He
    also discusses how many servings from each group should be eaten everyday.

Other Books to Read, Continued

MacDonald, E. (1990). <u>Mr</u>. <u>macgregor's</u> <u>breakfast</u> <u>egg</u>. New York: Penguin Group.
    As Mr. Cameron tries to deliver corn to Mr. MacGregor, a herd of cattle gets in his way. In
    front of the cattle is a group of boys on their bicycles and in front of them is a bus.
    Mr. MacGregor has to wait a long time for his corn.

McGovern, A. (1986). <u>Stone</u> <u>soup</u>. New York: Scholastic Inc.
    A young man is hungry and convinces an old woman that he can make soup from a stone.
    By the time the soup is ready, the woman has added several things from her garden to the
    soup. They eat the soup and when the boy leaves her house, he pulls the stone out of his pocket.

McMillan, B. (1989). <u>Time</u> <u>to</u>.... New York: Scholastic Inc.
    It is 7:00 a.m. and it is time to wake up. Breakfast is at 8:00 a.m. and school begins at
    9:00 a.m. After a long day, it is time to go to bed at 9:00 p.m.

Myers, B. (1990). <u>It</u> <u>happens</u> <u>to</u> <u>everyone</u>. New York: Lothrop, Lee and Shepard Books.
    It is the first day of school. Michael is nervous as he gets dressed, eats his breakfast, and
    rides the bus to school. Mrs. Daniels, a teacher, also gets ready for school. She is
    nervous, too.   When Michael and Mrs. Daniels arrive at school, they discover that they
    are in the same classroom.

Nikola-Lisa, W. (1991). <u>1,2,3 thanksgiving</u>. Morton Grove, IL: Albert Whitman & Company.
    It is Thanksgiving, so this book gives a step-by-step sequence of food preparations and how
    to set the table. It focuses on the numbers 1-8.

Novak, M. (1990). <u>Mr</u>. <u>floop's</u> <u>lunch</u>. New York: Orchard Books.
    Mr. Floop shares his lunch with animals in the park, but then Mr. Floop is hungry.
    A woman stops by and shares her lunch with Mr. Floop.

Richardson (1991). <u>Stephen's</u> <u>feast</u>. New York: Little, Brown and Company.
    Stephen, a page in King Wenceslas's court, is always being teased by other pages.
    Stephen is called upon to accompany the king on a journey through the snow and cold.
    Stephen is suprised to find out how enjoyable the trip is -- especially the feast at the end!

Robins, J. (1988). <u>Addie</u> <u>meets</u> <u>max</u>. New York: HarperCollins Children's Books.
    Addie is reluctant to befriend her new neighbor Max, especially after they run into each
    other when riding bikes. Addie's mom sets up a luncheon between the two of them, and
    they eventually become friends.

Other Books to Read,
Continued

Rockwell, H. (1980). My kitchen. New York: Greenwillow Books.
    The kitchen is a fun place work. There is a refrigerator where we keep food. There is a
    breadbox where we store bread. In the cupboards there are cans of soup, boxes of crackers,
    and treats!

Rylant, C. (1985). The relatives came. New York: Macmillan Children's Book Group.
    Relatives visit from Virginia with lots of laughter, hugs, food, and good times.
    During the reunion, they eat, sleep, and breathe together.

Shelby, A. (1991). Potluck. New York: Orchard Books.
    Alpha and Betty plan a potluck dinner and invite all their friends. Each person brings a
    different type of food. Acton brings asparagus, Ben brings bagels, Don brings dumplings
    and there are many more.

Viorst, J. (1987). Alexander and the terrible, horrible, no good, very bad day. New York: Scholastic Inc.
    Alexander has what everyone has experienced, a bad day. From gum in his hair in the
    morning to eating lima beans for dinner, nothing seems to go right the entire day. His mom
    tells him that there are days like that everywhere.

Watson, W. (1992). Hurray for the fourth of july. New York: Houghton Mifflin Co.
    A family shows how they enjoy celebrating the Fourth of July through a series of
    events like a parade, picnic, and watching fireworks.

Williams, B. (1978). Jeremy isn't hungry. New York: Dutton Children's Books.
    Davey tries to feed his difficult little brother, Jeremy, while his mom gets ready to go away.
    Davey tries many things, and finally Jeremy feeds himself.

Wood, A. (1987). Heckedy peg. San Diego: Scholastic Inc.
    A mother goes to market. While she is gone, a witch persuades her children to let her in the
    house. The witch turns the children into her supper, but the mother arrives home in time to save
    her children and chase the witch away.

Wynot, J. (1990). The mother's day sandwich. New York: Orchard Books.
    Ivy and Hackett decide to suprise their mom for Mother's Day by making her breakfast
    in bed. They make a real mess. When they wake up their mom, the food spills.
    She tells them she wants a hug (a Mother's Day Sandwich).

Focused Theme:
Markets, Bakeries, and Vendors

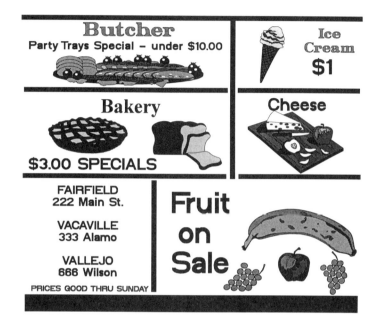

Overview of Markets, Bakeries, and Vendors:

This focused theme highlights three different places where we buy food to eat. Have you ever been to a large market or a mega grocery store? What do you like best about stopping at the bakery for your favorite bread or rolls? Have you ever bought any food on a street corner or roadside stand? The feature books in this section show what kinds of foods we buy when shopping, and the kinds of foods we make after getting home and unloading the grocery bags.

*Featured Book #1
of the Focused Theme:
Markets, Bakeries, and
Vendors*

My First Look at Shopping
edited by Andrea Pinnington
and Charlotte Davies
Random House, 1991

This lesson addresses the following Dietary Guidelines for Americans:

1. Eat a variety of foods.
2. Balance the food you eat with physical activity; maintain or improve your weight.
⇒ ***3. Choose a diet with plenty of grain products, vegetables, and fruits.***
4. Choose a diet low in fat, saturated fat, and cholesterol.
5. Choose a diet moderate in sugars.
6. Choose a diet moderate in salt and sodium.
7. Choose an alcohol and drug-free lifestyle.

This lesson highlights the following food groups from the Food Guide Pyramid:

⇒ ***Bread, Cereal, Rice, & Pasta Group***
⇒ ***Fruit Group***
⇒ ***Vegetable Group***
   Milk, Yogurt, & Cheese Group
   Meat, Poultry, Fish, Dry Beans, Eggs, & Nuts Group
⇒ ***Fats, Oils, and Sweets***

Food Guide Pyramid
A Guide to Daily Food Choices

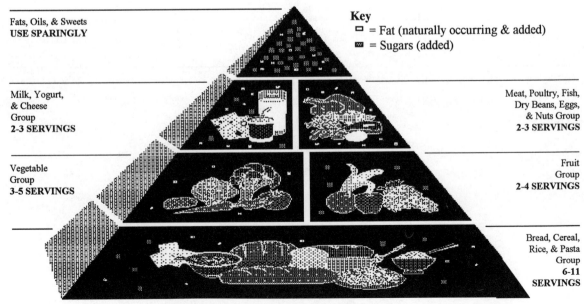

Fats, Oils, & Sweets
USE SPARINGLY

Key
□ = Fat (naturally occurring & added)
▨ = Sugars (added)

Milk, Yogurt,
& Cheese
Group
2-3 SERVINGS

Meat, Poultry, Fish,
Dry Beans, Eggs,
& Nuts Group
2-3 SERVINGS

Vegetable
Group
3-5 SERVINGS

Fruit
Group
2-4 SERVINGS

Bread, Cereal,
Rice, & Pasta
Group
**6-11
SERVINGS**

Source: U.S. Department of Agriculture & U.S. Department of Health and Human Services

Lesson Plans for Featured Book 1

Kindersley, D. (1991). <u>My</u> <u>first</u> <u>look</u> at <u>shopping</u>. New York: Random House, Inc.
There are many things people can buy when they go shopping. At the grocery,
there are apples, oranges, peppers, grapes, bananas, corn and lemons. At the bakery, there
is cake, croissants, fruit tarts, bread and pastries. There are many other stores to visit too.
Low reading level.

Pre-Reading Activities for *My First Look at Shopping*

Play the sequential memory game called "I'm going on a trip, A to Z". The game begins with one person
saying "I'm going to the grocery store and I'm going to buy some apples". The next person says: "I'm
going to the grocery store, and I'm going to buy some apples and bananas". The next person repeats the
sentence and adds on a food beginning with a letter C. Each person must repeat the previous foods in
alphabetical order then add a new selection which begins with the next letter of the alphabet. (MI = V/L,
M/R)

Post-Reading Activities for *My First Look at Shopping*

<u>Questions to develop thinking skills</u> (Bloom's Taxonomy)

1. Knowledge: Count and name the different places where we can go shopping.

2. Comprehension: Recognize which two places in the book have food shopping.

3. Application: Collect magazine pictures of foods from the bakery and foods from the
greengrocer's. Keep the pictures in two separate classroom boxes for later
use.

4. Analysis: Categorize each of the foods sold at the bakery (from the book) into one or
more food groups from the Food Guide Pyramid.

5. Synthesis: Change the name of the greengrocer's to another word or words that we
might use to describe a place that sells fruits and vegetables.

6. Evaluation: Recommend another section of the book which could show other
foods for sale. For example, a meat market. What other food stores
can you think of?

Solo Work for *My First Look at Shopping*

Write and illustrate a short story that explains a shopping trip you took with a friend or family member. (MI = V/L, V/S)

Small Group Work for *My First Look at Shopping*

In groups of three to four students, look at mail catalogs that sell food. How does the food look in the pictures? Does it appeal to your visual senses? Can you imagine what it tastes like? Feels like? Smells like? Write a description of one of the foods in the catalog using adjectives that captures your senses. Advertise the food in a mock radio or television commercial. Share both the written advertisement and verbal advertisement with your class. (MI = V/S, B/K, V/L, I/S)

Whole Class Work for *My First Look at Shopping*

Malls have become large social centers for shopping, exercising, eating, and gathering to talk. How many malls are in your community? What are their names? What grocery stores are found at the four-corner crossroads nearest the malls? Do you see any trends or patterns from mall to mall? As a class, make a large map of your community showing where the malls and major grocery stores are located. If you are from a smaller community without a mall, make your map so it shows the major grocery stores. (MI = V/L)

Divide your class into teams to do the following.
1) Contact the Chamber of Commerce in your community to see if they have a shopping guide of your area. Request a few copies for your classroom.
2) Contact your local newspaper to see if they have any shopping guides of your area.
3) Contact a local Realtor to see if they have any shopping guides of your area.
4) Contact one of the largest super stores in your area which serves as both a grocery store and a department store. Request a couple maps showing the inside layout of the store. Are the two sections of the store similar in size?
5) Contact one of the grocery store chains in your area. Request a floor plan of the store, so you can see where different foods are organized in the store. How many grocery stores in your area also have a restaurant inside?
6) Make a list of specialized food shops that exist in your community. For example, bagel shops, bakeries, candy stores, meat markets, produce markets, yogurt shops, and ice cream shops. These specialized food shops are places where you can buy a certain kind of food to take home. Yogurt and ice cream shops can also be a restaurant to its customers who wish to eat there too.

Before you start the steps above, complete a KWWWL chart (Gonser & Burz, 1991) as a class. Each component of the chart is explained below:
K =   What do we know? (prior knowledge)
W =   What do we need or want to know? (key questions by students and teachers)
W =   Where are we going to find out? (resources, technology, research)
W =   What are we going to do with our information, findings, new questions? (outcomes, sharing)
L =   What have we learned? (assessment, student outcomes)

Use your findings in this "shopping study" to prepare you for the next two feature books in this unit.

Across the Curriculum for *My First Look at Shopping*

Social Studies

When were mega markets first introduced? Compare the history of mega markets, shopping malls, and strip malls (plaza shopping). (MI = V/L)

Mathematics

Most fresh foods are sold by weight. Using a food scale, weigh different amounts of produce. Look in the local grocery advertisements to see how much the food costs per pound. Calculate how much your food will cost based on its weight. (MI = L/M)

Science

Today many of our foods are purchased already canned or frozen from a grocery store. Some people still preserve their garden foods by freezing them or canning them. Canned foods are then stored in a place that is cool and dry. Canning is a very good way to keep foods from spoiling. Investigate how canning is done in home kitchens. Why is canning both a science and an art? (MI = V/L)

Language Arts

Buy a magazine at a grocery check-out counter or bring an old magazine from home. Count the number of articles about food or eating in the magazine. Make a list of the titles. Compare your list with another person who chose another type of magazine. (MI = L/M, I/S)

Physical Education

Mall walking is a very popular form of exercise in many communities. How do you know how far you are walking in a mall? Have you ever exercised (walk, jogged, hiked) with a pedometer? Using a pedometer, walk the hallways of your school until you have traveled one-half mile. Also notice the time it took for you to walk the half mile. Make a chart showing the distance and time of your walk for three days. Try to keep up your exercise plan for a couple weeks. What changes do you see from week to week? (MI = B/K, L/M, I/I)

Art

Design a floor plan for a new grocery store in your community. What foods would you put at the perimeter of the store and what foods would you put close to the checkout? Label your floor plan with careful lettering, and be sure to include a key for your floor plan. Also have a contest to design the store sign which discloses the new name of the grocery store. (MI = V/S, V/L)

Music

Sing the Raffi song called "The Corner Grocery Store" (See the Teaching Resources at the back of the book). Sing the song with the recording for a while, then try to sing it without musical accompaniment (acappella). (MI = M/R)

Across the Curriculum

---

*Featured Book #2
of the Focused Theme:
Markets, Bakeries, and
Vendors*

Walter the Baker
by Eric Carle
Simon & Schuster Books for
Young Readers, 1995

This lesson addresses the following Dietary Guidelines for Americans:

1. Eat a variety of foods.
2. Balance the food you eat with physical activity; maintain or improve your weight.
⇒   *3. Choose a diet with plenty of grain products, vegetables, and fruits.*
4. Choose a diet low in fat, saturated fat, and cholesterol.
⇒   *5. Choose a diet moderate in sugars.*
⇒   *6. Choose a diet moderate in salt and sodium.*
7. Choose an alcohol and drug-free lifestyle.

This lesson highlights the following food groups from the Food Guide Pyramid:

⇒   *Bread, Cereal, Rice, & Pasta Group*
Fruit Group
Vegetable Group
⇒   *Milk, Yogurt, & Cheese Group*
Meat, Poultry, Fish, Dry Beans, Eggs, & Nuts Group

Food Guide Pyramid
A Guide to Daily Food Choices

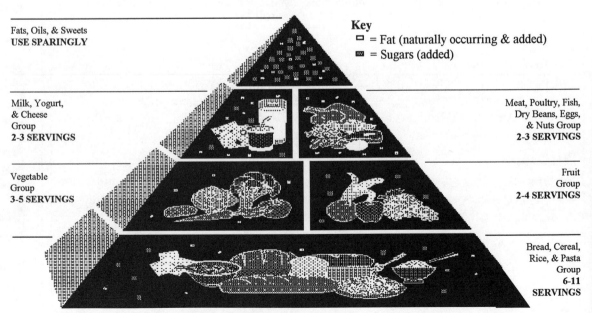

Source: U.S. Department of Agriculture & U.S. Department of Health and Human Services

Lesson Plans to Featured Book 2

Carle, E. (1995). <u>Walter the baker</u>. New York: Simon & Schuster Books for Young Readers.
The Duke and Duchess love the sweet rolls prepared by Walter the Baker each morning.
One morning, an accident forces Walter to change his recipe which results in a bad tasting
sweet roll. In order to stay in the kingdom, the Duke orders Walter to create "a roll
through which the rising sun can shine three times, be made from one piece of dough, and
taste good". In his effort to please the Duke and Duchess, and to prevent being banished
from his homeland, Walter creates the pretzel. Advanced reading level.

Pre-Reading Activities for *Walter the Baker*

Visit a local bakery. How big do you think a bakery oven is? How many different kinds of bakery
products are there? Ask to see some of the following baked goods: strudle, tarts, scones, muffins,
sweetrolls, elephant ears, doughnuts, bagels, pita, rolls, and biscuits. Which baked goods are made with
the same recipe but are baked differently? (MI = V/L)

Post-Reading Activities for *Walter the Baker*

Questions to develop thinking skills (Bloom's Taxonomy)

1. Knowledge: List the events that resulted in Walter inventing the pretzel.

2. Comprehension: Restate the criteria for the roll Walter had to make in order to remain a citizen
of Duchy.

3. Application: Report the news to the local town crier of Duchy that a pretzel has been created.
Be sure to include the name of the creator and the steps he took to create this new
food.

4. Analysis: Examine the foods that the Duke and Duchess were eating in story. What
food groups of the food pyramid did they leave out?

5. Synthesis: Improve Walter's work plan now that he has another roll to bake in the morning.
Create a work plan so that Walter does not lose any sleep. You may also include
other characters.

6. Evaluation: Which characters do you consider healthier, Walter and his wife or the Duke and
Duchess? Defend your opinion with details from the story and your own life
experiences.

Solo Work for *Walter the Baker*

Walter used his creativity and problem solving ability to invent a tasty roll "through which the rising sun can shine three times". In your opinion, what was the most interesting thing about Walter's efforts? What kind of work ethics and work style did he model? What happened when another person, e.g., his son, took a look at the problem? Who else assisted in the final product? Think of a time in your life when working together as a team produced a better product. Make a picture of the product that resulted. Write a caption for your product then display it on the wall. Please put your initials on the front of the picture in the bottom right hand corner. (MI = V/L, V/S, I/S)

Small Group Work for *Walter the Baker*

In small groups of three to four students, read the book aloud one more time. Pass the book from person to person in your group so that each of you has a chance to read aloud. Next complete a Story Web as a group. A story web includes the title of the book, the author of the book, the setting of the story, names of the main characters, the problem, and the solution. Compare your answers with one other small group in your class. (MI = V/L, V/S, I/S)

Whole Class Work for *Walter the Baker*

Each person should remove one picture from the wall that does not belong to you. Study the picture of the product and think about the caption. How can you modify or improve the product as shown? Write a few ideas on the back of the picture. Exchange papers with another person in class without talking. Again, study the picture of the product and think about the caption. How can you modify or improve the product as shown? Continue the exchange of papers and reflective brainstorming for five more rotations. Return the picture to the wall.

Next, remove your picture from the wall that has your initials on it. Take a few moments to look at the ideas that your classmates wrote on the back of your paper. Some ideas will seem very silly, some ideas may seem somewhat strange, and usually one idea (and sometimes more) will really seem to be instructive, original, and/or interesting. Listen to some thinking music as a class while focusing and concentrating on the one idea that you liked. Let your mind wander and be creative as you look for connections between your original product and the new idea. What new product or idea results? Write a paragraph about how you tried a new way of thinking.

Finally, as a class, do some creative problem solving about a food or nutrition problem at your school. Use your new ways of thinking to come up with a different product or a different idea. Talk with your school Food Service Director about one or two problems that exist in the cafeteria. What can your class do to make a difference and improve the current situation? Don't forget to share your experiences with your local newspaper, radio station, and/or television station. (MI = V/L, I/S)

Across the Curriculum for *Walter the Baker*
Social Studies

Research the royal lines that have formed the government for many countries. What are the responsibilities of a King, Queen, Duke, Duchess, Baron, Baroness, Earl (Count), Countess, Prince, and Princess? Many bakery products come from different countries. Did you know that some products are even named for the country's leaders, such as Napoleons or kringles? Investigate the different kinds of pastries and their origins. Consider having a tea party where you take on the roles of different nobility as you enjoy eating different pastries. (MI = V/L, B/K)

Mathematics

Pretzels come in many different shapes and sizes. Some pretzels are thin and straight and some are thick and straight.Other pretzels are shaped as nuggets, rounds, wagonwheels, and combos. Sort a variety of pretzels by size and shape. Use the pretzels as manipulatives to solve math equations. Be sure you save a few pretzels on the side that won't get handled as manipulatives by you or others. Destination? Your belly! Pretzels are a delicious, low-fat food for snacks and parties. (MI = L/M, B/K)

Science

Most breads require a leavening agent to make them rise. Place one package of yeast, 1/2 cup of sugar, 1 cup of flour, and 1 cup of warm water into a flask or a container with a narrow top. Mix and stir the ingredients. Place a balloon over the top of the flask. As the yeast works, the balloon will fill with air. Investigate the leavening agent for quick breads, e.g., baking powder and cream of tartar. (MI = B/K)

Language Arts

Read the author's notes in the back of *Walter the Baker*. Many of our English words like pretzel comes from Latin. What other names of foods are derived from Latin? Make a list of food words in English with their Latin etymology. Etymology? What's that? Look in a dictionary to learn more. Have you ever noticed the number of pages in a dictionary that gives information about language? There's more to a dictionary than definitions and correct spellings. Compare different dictionaries as you look for different food words and their history. (MI = V/L)

Physical Education

Make a human pretzel in groups of five or six students. Form a circle and hold hands. One student reaches across the circle to grasp the hand of another student. Do not grasp the hand of the person to the left or right of you. Without losing grip with the two students in your group, try to untangle the pretzel. This activity develops your spatial awareness, balance, and flexibility. (MI = B/K)

Art

Build a medieval castle or village like the Duke and Duchess lived in by using food cartons and packaging for the buildings. Hold pretzels together by peanut butter or clay to make simple structures. Blue gelatin on a mirror or glass makes a good moat or pond. What other food products and packaging will you use? (MI = V/S, B/K)

Music

Play songs that still exist from medieval times, e.g., *Greensleeves (What Child is This?)* and *Good King Wenceslaus,* during your tea party or art activities. (MI = M/R)

Across the Curriculum

113

Featured Book #3 of the Focused Theme: Markets, Bakeries, and Vendors	# *Frannie's Fruits* # by Leslie Kimmelman # HarperCollins Children's Books, # 1989

This lesson addresses the following Dietary Guidelines for Americans:

⇒   *1. Eat a variety of foods.*

     2. Balance the food you eat with physical activity; maintain or improve your weight.

⇒   *3. Choose a diet with plenty of grain products, vegetables, and fruits.*

     4. Choose a diet low in fat, saturated fat, and cholesterol.

     5. Choose a diet moderate in sugars.

     6. Choose a diet moderate in salt and sodium.

     7. Choose an alcohol and drug-free lifestyle.

This lesson highlights the following food groups from the Food Guide Pyramid:

     Bread, Cereal, Rice, & Pasta Group

⇒   *Fruit Group*

⇒   *Vegetable Group*

     Milk, Yogurt, & Cheese Group

     Meat, Poultry, Fish, Dry Beans, Eggs, & Nuts Group

Food Guide Pyramid
A Guide to Daily Food Choices

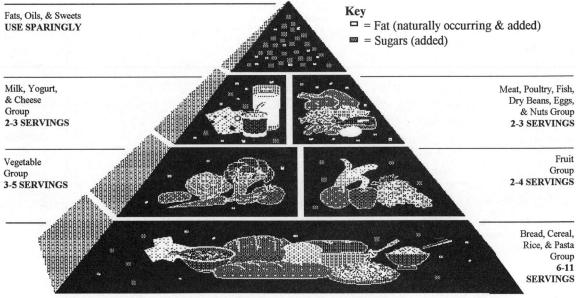

Source: U.S. Department of Agriculture & U.S. Department of Health and Human Services

Lesson Plans for Featured Book 3

Kimmelman, L. (1989). <u>Frannie's fruits</u>. New York: HarperCollins Children's Books.
A little girl and her family operate a fruit and vegetable stand near the beach with
the help of their dog, Frannie. She enjoys seeing all the different customers come into
buy different things. Intermediate reading level.

Pre-Reading Activities for *Frannie's Fruits*

Describe a time when your family stopped by an outdoor food market. Was it by the ocean? In the country? On the sidewalk in a city? Or another place? Describe some of the sights and sounds you remember from your outing. Why do the vendors cover up their foods and goods at the end of the day? What is the purpose of the tent awnings and roofs overhead during the day when the market is full of activity? (MI = V/L)

Post-Reading Activities for *Frannie's Fruits*

<u>Questions to develop thinking skills</u> (Bloom's Taxonomy)

1. *Knowledge:*   Name some of the various items sold at the family stand. Were they all fruits?

2. *Comprehension:* Restate the different events that happened at the stand during one day.

3. *Application:*   Role play a character from the story that you like. Experiment with different dialects.

4. *Analysis:*   Categorize the items sold at Frannie's Fruits. What areas of the food pyramid are not covered at this stand? What items are not part of the food pyramid?

5. *Synthesis:*   What if the narrator's family owned a butcher shop? Imagine the ways her life would be different.

6. *Evaluation:*   Judge whether people working at Frannie's Fruits are physically fit. Revise one person's schedule so he or she could stretch to get more flexibility during the day.

Solo Work for *Frannie's Fruits*

Make a food puppet out of a fruit or vegetable. Use drinking straws, pipe cleaners, and popsicle sticks for arms and legs. Use raisins, seeds, nuts, and candy for other body parts. Use alliteration to name your puppet, e.g., Buster Banana, Paulina Pepper, or Courtney Carrot. (MI = B/K, V/L)

Small Group Work for *Frannie's Fruits*

Group students by the type of food puppet they made. For example, put all the bananas together and all the potatoes together. Investigate the nutrient value of the food and write a short script for each character to share with the class. Use the name of each puppet when introducing new food information. "Hi, I'm Otto Orange, and I am a tropical fruit that is rich in Vitamin C". "Hi, I'm Opal Orange, and I can give you all the Vitamin C your body needs in one day. Just squeeze me into orange juice and take a drink!" (MI = B/K, V/L)

Whole Class Work for *Frannie's Fruits*

Perform your small group skits for the entire class. Discuss a way for all the skits to be adapted into a larger skit or production. Some students might be chosen to be a narrator or other human characters. For example, the greengrocer could say, "I just received this shipment of lemons from Arizona". He opens the box and a lemon puppet pops out. A student controlling the lemon puppet could say "It was a long trip, but I still have lots of vitamin C. I, Leslie Lemon, would be happy to be a cool lemonade drink for you on his hot, sunny day." When planning your skit, investigate where the different foods come from by looking at the pictures in the story for assistance. For example, there are "Needlessly Seedless Grapes" from California and Long Island Potatoes.

The entire class can work together to build the scenery or set for the production. The setting is a market or group of vendor stands where customers gather to purchase produce. Deliveries and shipment can be coming and going from across the country and all over the world. Use different languages and a variety of geographical maps and flags wherever appropriate in the storyline. Be sure to share food and nutrition information so your audience learns not only what foods are nutritious to eat, but where food comes from and how it gets to markets and vendors for us to buy. (MI = B/K, V/L, V/S, I/S)

Across the Curriculum for *Frannie's Fruits*

Social Studies

Look in the book to see the interactions of people with different animals. Research the social relationship that people have enjoyed with animals. Talk about how we socialize with animals and how animals often respond to our emotions and actions. For example, a loud child can be quieted when petting a rabbit or a cat. (MI = V/L)

Mathematics

Produce is packaged and sold in different quantities. Investigate the differences in quantity and price between a quart, a peck, and a bushel of food. Foods may also be sold by the dozen (bakers dozen), by the piece, or by the pound. Find examples for each of these quantities by visiting a roadside stand, a farmer's market, or grocery store. Can't go there today? Compare the prices of different fruits and vegetables in the story. Which are more expensive and which are the least expensive? (MI = L/M)

Science

Fresh and dried flowers are often sold at markets, because their colors and fragrance often appeals to customers when shopping. Have you ever made a dried flower arrangement? To dry flowers, place their stems into holes of some hanging chicken wire. Within a couple weeks, the flowers will be ready to be arranged into baskets or vases. Also experiment with drying fruit in a food dehydrator. Weigh the food before and after it is dried. The difference in the weight is the loss of water. (MI = B/K, V/S, L/M)

Language Arts

Look at the pictures in the story for questionable safety practices. For example a knife, scissors, and a trowel are left on an open table in the market. Other examples are open fertilizer on the table, cat left in a hot car, boy running while eating a banana, ear phones with music too loud, and riding in an open truck bed. Write several sentences on how one of the unsafe situations could be made safer in the story. (MI = V/L)

Physical Education

Form a "people chain" for passing objects down a line over a long distance. For example, people chains are used when sandbags are moved into place to form a dike against a flood or when crates need to be unloaded from a truck. Repetitive movements of your arms and legs will increase your muscular endurance. Have you ever felt your muscle get tired after you lifted the same thing over and over again? Use a people chain next time so you can get twice as much moved with less effort. You will still need to practice lifting with your muscles a couple times a week, so they can adapt to the workload and gradually get stronger. (MI = B/K)

Art

Puppets are an old art form. The ancient Persians and Siamese used a form of puppets on a reflection screen to tell stories. Study the art of puppet making and use different mediums (e.g., paper mache) for making a puppet. (MI = V/L, V/S)

Music

Does music make it easier to perform a "people chain". Try it and see for yourself! (MI = B/K, M/R)

Across the Curriculum

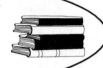

*Other Books to Read for
"Markets, Bakeries, and
Vendors"*

This list contains excellent books to read for learning about Markets, Bakeries, and Vendors. Use these books along with the Featured Books when teaching the lessons on the previous pages.

Brooks, B. (1991). Lemonade parade. Morton Grove, IL: Albert Whitman & Company.
    In summer, a few young children set up a lemonade stand. A father dresses up as
    different customers so the children will earn money.

Budd, L. (1960). The pie wagon. New York: Lothrop, Lee and Shepard Books.
    A pie man sells pies to the people of a town. A little girl chooses a pie from a selection labeled
    A to Z. The pie wagon goes onto the next town.

Cohen, P. & L. O. (1989). Olson's meat pies. New York: R & S Books.
    Olson makes meat pies with the best ingredients. One day Olson's bookkeeper runs off
    with all of his money. Olson is forced to put strange ingredients in the pies -- like
    watches. When the bookkeeper comes back with most of Olson's money, the meat
    pies are good again.

Czernecki, S., & Rhodes, T. (1992). The sleeping bread. New York: Hyperion Paperbacks for Children.
    Beto is a breadmaker who becomes friends with Zafiro, the town beggar. The townspeople
    ask Zafiro to leave because they are embarrassed by him. When Beto's bread does not rise,
    they find Zafiro to help Beto's bread rise again.

de Regniers, B. S. (1987). The snow party. New York: Lothrop, Lee and Shepard Books.
    A lonely husband and wife live alone. When a big snowstorm hits, many people
    become stranded, so they ask if they can stay at the couple's house. The couple enjoys
    the company of the people, and they have a huge party.

Feder, P. K. (1992). Where does the teacher live? New York: Dutton Children's Books.
    Alba, Willie, and Nancy are all students in Mrs. Greengrass's class. They all wonder
    where their teacher lives and search for several days. They watch her walk out of
    school each day and collected clues. They finally ask Mrs. Greengrass where
    she lives. She rewards them with ice cream cones for being such good detectives.

Forest, H. (1993). The bakers dozen. San Diego: Harcourt Brace & Co.
    Jan Van Amsterdam is a well known baker. People travel from all over to buy his goods.
    When he begins to get greedy, he starts to use less ingredients in his cookies. When a
    woman asks for a bakers dozen, he only gives her 12. She puts a curse on him and his
    baked goods. When he realizes that a bakers dozen is 13, the curse is broken.

Other Books to Read,
Continued

Garland, S. (1982). <u>Going shopping</u>. London: Bodley Head Ltd.
>   A family goes grocery shopping. They buy food, pack it up, and then drive home again.

Greeson, J. (1952). <u>The stingy baker</u>. Minneapolis: Carolrhoda Books, Inc.
>   Jan is a stingy baker. When a woman enters his cookie shop and asks for a bakers
>   dozen, Jan refuses to give her an extra free cookie. The woman puts an evil spell on Jan.
>   When Jan finally gives her a bakers dozen of cookies, the spell is broken.

Hutchins, P. (1989). <u>Don't forget the bacon</u>. New York: William Morrow & Co., Inc.
>   A boy is sent to the store for bacon and other groceries. As the boy walks to the store, he
>   repeats over and over what he is supposed to get. He becomes thoroughly confused and
>   forgets about the bacon. Once he gets home, he is sent back for the bacon.

Krockover, G., & Krockover, S. (1978). <u>Uncle bill's ice cream shop</u>. New York: Vantage Press.
>   A girl talks about her Uncle Bill's Ice Cream Shop. She describes the different kinds of
>   ice cream and tells of her favorite flavors.

Lakin, P. (1994). <u>Don't forget</u>. New York: William Morrow & Company Inc.
>   Sarah shares secrets with her neighbors, the Singers, who are Holocaust
>   survivors. She talks with them while out shopping for ingredients for her mother's birthday. For
>   example, an orange, cake flour, baking powder, sugar, and eggs are part of the birthday surprise.

Levitin (1980). <u>Nobody stole the pie</u>. San Diego: Harcourt Brace & Co.
>   In the town of Little Digby, there is a Lollyberry tree that grows delicious berries. Each
>   year, they have a festival and eat a big lollyberry pie. Everyone takes a little piece
>   throughout the day and thinks nothing of it. By the time of the celebration, there is only one
>   piece left for the mayor. Nobody admits to stealing the pie, but the mayor knows
>   everybody stole the pie.

Lobel, A. (1989). <u>On market street</u>. New York: Scholastic Inc.
>   A little boy goes to the market to buy gifts for his friend. He buys gifts that begin with each
>   letter of the alphabet. The market is rich with colorful foods.

Newcome, Z. (1991). <u>Rosie goes shopping</u>. London: Julia MacRae Books.
>   Rosie and her mother go on a shopping trip. They buy many different foods and other
>   needed items.

Other Books to Read,
Continued

Salt, J., & Hawksley, G. (1990). <u>First words and pictures</u>. New York: Larousse Kingfisher Chambers.
A baby has many new things to see and touch at the supermarket. At home, it is time to unload the groceries and make dinner.

Sendak, M. (1970). <u>In the night kitchen</u>. New York: HarperCollins Children's Books.
In his dream, Mickey falls out of bed into the batter of cake in the kitchen. He goes through many obstacles to help the bakers get the milk they need for their cake.

Van Leeuwen, J. (1974). <u>Too hot for ice cream</u>. New York: Dial Books For Young Readers.
On their way to the park, Elizabeth and Sarah stop to buy ice cream. However, it is such a hot day that the ice cream melts all over them. Before they make it to the park, it begins to rain so they decide to turn around and go back home.

Wellington, M. (1992). <u>Mr. cookie baker</u>. New York: Dutton Children's Books.
Mr. Baker enjoys making, decorating, selling, and eating his cookies.

Williams, J. (1992). <u>Playtime 123</u>. New York: Dial Books For Young Readers.
Counting to 20 can be fun! Nine children go on a Sunday picnic and 10 bear-buddies eat in the sun. Later on in this book, 19 children run to the ice cream truck and eat a treat.

Yorinks, A. (1986). <u>Louis the fish</u>. New York: Farrar, Straus, & Giroux.
Louis inherits his father's meat store after he dies. Louis never liked meat before and prefers fish. He eventually turns into a fish himself.

Focused Theme:
Diners, Restaurants, and Soup Kitchens

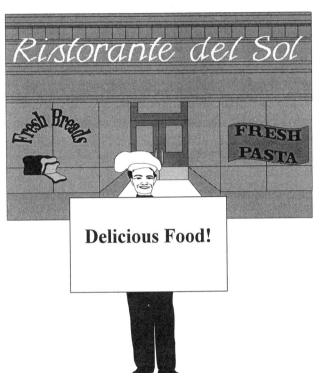

<u>Overview of Diners, Restaurants, and Soup Kitchens:</u>

This focused theme emphasizes eating behavior in three different public places where food is eaten. Eating behavior is designated by *what* we eat, *when* we eat, *where* we eat, and *with whom* we eat. What food do you eat at your favorite restaurant? Do you like to go with anyone in particular? Do you tend to eat more food or less food when you go out to eat? This section will highlight where we eat. The feature books in this section also address what kinds of foods and with whom we eat our meals.

---

*Featured Book #1
of the Focused Theme:
Diners, Restaurants, and
Soup Kitches*

In the Diner
by Christine Loomis
Scholastic Inc., 1994

This lesson addresses the following Dietary Guidelines for Americans:

1. Eat a variety of foods.
2. Balance the food you eat with physical activity; maintain or improve your weight.
3. Choose a diet with plenty of grain products, vegetables, and fruits.
⇒ *4. Choose a diet low in fat, saturated fat, and cholesterol.*
⇒ *5. Choose a diet moderate in sugars.*
6. Choose a diet moderate in salt and sodium.
7. Choose an alcohol and drug-free lifestyle.

This lesson highlights the following food groups from the Food Guide Pyramid:

⇒ *Bread, Cereal, Rice, & Pasta Group*
Fruit Group
Vegetable Group
⇒ *Milk, Yogurt, & Cheese Group*
⇒ *Meat, Poultry, Fish, Dry Beans, Eggs, & Nuts Group*
⇒ *Fats, Oils, & Sweets*

Food Guide Pyramid
A Guide to Daily Food Choices

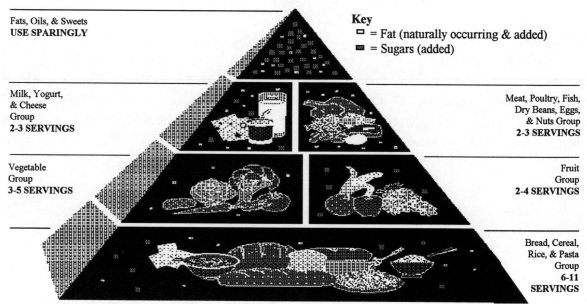

Source: U.S. Department of Agriculture & U.S. Department of Health and Human Services

Lesson Plans for Featured Book 1

Loomis, C. (1994). In the diner. New York: Scholastic Inc.
The diner is a busy place. Waiters run around, busboys set the tables, and chefs prepare the food. Bacon sizzles, coffee brews, bagels toast, burgers broil, and many other things happen in the busy diner. Low reading level.

Pre-Reading Activities for *In the Diner*

Write names of different foods from the story on flashcards. Hand a flashcard to each student and have them read the word then say how the food sounds. For example, bacon sizzles, carrots crunch, and soup slurps. (MI = V/L)

Use a yellow pages phone book to see how many diners are in your community. Write them on the board. Take a class vote to see how many students have ever eaten in the different diners. What is the difference between a diner and a fast food restaurant? (MI = V/L, L/M)

Post-Reading Activities for *In the Diner*

Questions to develop thinking skills (Bloom's Taxonomy)

1. *Knowledge:* List and label the different workers in the diner.

2. *Comprehension:* Draw a sequence picture showing the events of the day at the diner.

3. *Application:* Collect pairs of action verbs from the story. Experiment with new verbs to tell the story.

4. *Analysis:* Categorize the foods served at the diner into the five food groups. Could a customer order a well-balanced meal at this diner? Give supporting details.

5. *Synthesis:* Imagine the various conversations in the diner during one day. What might the customers be saying about the food, the workers, and the atmosphere?

6. *Evaluation:* Decide if this diner is a nutritious, safe, and clean restaurant. Give supporting details for each. What letter grade would give this diner? Why?

Solo Work for *In the Diner*

Choose a character from the book. Read the story again and see what the person does from page to page. Did you select a leading role or supporting role in the story? Give yourself a name as an actor or actress in this story. Do you eat in the story or help others eat in the story? (MI = I/I, V/L)

Small Group Work for *In the Diner*

With a group of two or three students, write a new story or skit that takes place at a diner. What's the name of your diner? What's your leading meal? Is your diner known best for its breakfasts, lunches, or dinners? Has anyone famous ever eaten at your diner? What do your characters wear at the diner? What music is played at the diner? Plan your story right down to the color of your tablecloths and placemats. What props will you need to carry out your ideas? (MI = I/S, V/L, V/S)

Whole Class Work for *In the Diner*

Set up your classroom to resemble a diner. Each group will practice their story or skit. Take turns working as the director, who calls for the sound stick or movie clapper. Will you play music during your skit? Videotape the different skits called "Dinner at the Diner" or "Lunch at the Luncheonette". Will any of your skits get a nomination for an Academy Award? Don't forget to award points to the diner with the most nutritious food. Use the Food Guide Pyramid to help you determine extra Fats, Oils, and Sweets in the different menus. (MI = V/S, V/L, I/S, L/M, M/R)

Across the Curriculum for *In the Diner*
Social Studies
Diners originated on trains. As people traveled across the country, people still had to eat their meals. The diner cars were busy, loud places to eat. Some famous trains include the Orient Express and the Flying Dutchman. As long-distance trains rides gave way to automobile travel, diners moved from trains to towns. Some more recent movies which depict diners on trains include "Murder on the Orient Express", "Trains of India", and "Fried Green Tomatoes". Read about diner trains and see how they compare to diners in your community. (MI = V/L)

Mathematics
Count the number of women, men, and children that enter the diner in the story. How many are school-aged children, and how many are elderly? What other categories can you use for counting the people in the story? (MI = L/M)

Science
Investigate how a drinking straw works. Experiment with different types of beverages like water, soda, milk shake, and tomato soup? Can you suck Jell-o through a straw? Some restaurants use a wider straw for their different beverages. How does the diameter of a straw effect the ability to suck the beverage into your mouth? (MI = B/K, L/M)

Language Arts
Write sentences from the book on paper at an easel board. Cut the sentences apart, and hand a paper strip to each student. Students should cut the sentences so they have individual word cards. Place all words in a basket and shuffle them. Each student then chooses two word cards from the basket and tries to complete a sentence by working with their classmates. Try to do this one card at a time. When a complete sentence is found, students can identify the number of syllables, vowels, or silent sounds in the sentence. (MI = V/L, I/S)

Physical Education
How many miles does a waitress, waiter, or bus boy walk during a shift? Experiment with a pedometer in the classroom. Practice carrying plates and trays like servers in a restaurant. Add a book on your tray. How about a book and a notebook? Or two plates? How is your coordination and balance while walking with a tray? Does your arm get tired holding it in one position? How does your arm feel? What kind of shoes should you wear while doing this activity? (Skills developed: coordination, balance, agility, static endurance). (MI = B/K)

Art
Create a menu card for your diner. Be sure to use a food pyramid on each menu to help people eating at the diner to choose a variety of food in moderation. Experiment with the use of primary colors (red, yellow, and blue) to code foods as "Eat Anytime", "Eat in Moderation", and "Eat Occasionally" on the menu card. (MI = V/S)

Music
Study the history of a juke box for playing records in public places. Play and compare music in your classroom from records, cassette tapes, and compact disks. (MI = M/R)

Across the Curriculum

Featured Book #2 of the Focused Theme: Diners, Restaurants, and Soup Kitchens

Pizza for Breakfast
by Maryann Kovalski
Morrow Junior Books, 1990

This lesson addresses the following Dietary Guidelines for Americans:

1. Eat a variety of foods.
2. Balance the food you eat with physical activity; maintain or improve your weight.
⇒ 3. *Choose a diet with plenty of grain products, vegetables, and fruits.*
⇒ 4. *Choose a diet low in fat, saturated fat, and cholesterol.*
5. Choose a diet moderate in sugars.
⇒ 6. *Choose a diet moderate in salt and sodium.*
7. Choose an alcohol and drug-free lifestyle.

This lesson highlights the following food groups from the Food Guide Pyramid:

⇒ *Bread, Cereal, Rice, & Pasta Group*
⇒ *Fruit Group*
   Vegetable Group
⇒ *Milk, Yogurt, & Cheese Group*
⇒ *Meat, Poultry, Fish, Dry Beans, Eggs, & Nuts Group*

Food Guide Pyramid
A Guide to Daily Food Choices

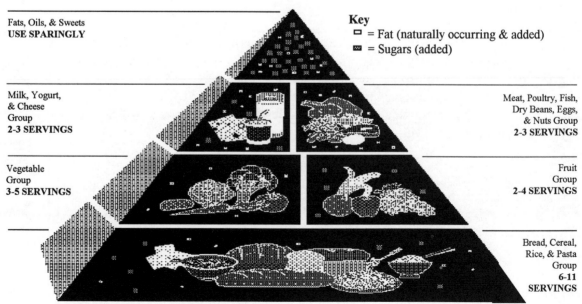

Source: U.S. Department of Agriculture & U.S. Department of Health and Human Services

Lesson Plans for Featured Book 2

Kovalski, M. (1990). <u>Pizza</u> <u>for</u> <u>breakfast</u>. New York: Morrow Junior Books.
Frank and Zeldo own a pizza place. When business gets slow, a strange man appears and
grants them wishes. The pizza place is soon booming and is too much for them to handle.
They decide to try something new so they move to the beach and set up a pizza stand.
Intermediate reading level.

Pre-Reading Activities for *Pizza for Breakfast*

Discuss what chores or work-related activities make you really tired. For example, raking leaves in the
Fall, scrubbing the bathtub, sweeping the sidewalk, or vacuuming the floors. Pantomime the
movements and let your classmates guess what you are doing by asking questions. (MI =B/K, V/L, I/S)

Talk about the type of food you usually eat for breakfast. Where does the food fit on the food pyramid?
What was the most unusal food you have ever had for breakfast? Have you ever had pizza for
breakfast? (MI = V/L, I/I)

Post-Reading Activities for *Pizza for Breakfast*

<u>Questions to develop thinking skills</u> (Bloom's Taxonomy)

1. *Knowledge:* Write the reasons why the people stopped coming to Frank and Zelda's for pizza.

2. *Comprehension:* Explain how Frank and Zelda's attitudes changed during the story.

3. *Application:* Put in order a list of suggestions that Frank and Zelda might give to people
   starting their own restaurant business.

4. *Analysis:* Examine Frank and Zelda's final business choice. Was this a healthful choice for
   the two them at this time? Why or why not?

5. *Synthesis:* What if Frank and Zelda would not have received help from the waiters when they
   were extremely busy? What do you imagine would have happened to Frank, Zelda,
   and their restaurant?

6. *Evaluation:* Argue for or against the choice of having pizza for breakfast. Give strong
   supporting details for the side you choose.

Solo Work for *Pizza for Breakfast*

Each student will weave a placemat using the back page of the book, *Pizza for Breakfast*, as a pattern. Once the placemat is made, trace around a paper plate in the middle of your placemat so that create a pizza. Decorate your pizza with cut out vegetables and cheese. Perhaps you can laminate your placemat with clear contact paper so you use it during your all-class pizza party. (MI = V/S)

Small Group Work for *Pizza for Breakfast*

Small groups of three or four students will make a grocery list for a salad bar at the all-class pizza party. Another group of students can help to determine what low-fat and low-cost salad dressings to have available at the all-class pizza party. Another group of students can investigate how many of the pizza restaurants in your community have sit-down dining inside the restaurants. Another group of students can investigate how many of the pizza restaurants have a delivery service and what the service costs. (MI = V/L, I/S, L/M)

Whole Class Work for *Pizza for Breakfast*

Based on the information gathered during your small group work, determine what pizza vendor in your community might be interested in hosting a class field trip to their restaurant or in donating pizza to the classroom for an all-class pizza party. Use a speaker phone in your classroom to call a few of these vendors to determine their interest and availability. Your school food service could even supply the pizza for an all-class party if prior arrangements are made for funding and availability. After the meal, talk to the owner of the pizza restaurant about how the business is operated and the effects of a restaurant business on personal and family time. (MI = V/L, B/K, L/M)

Across the Curriculum for *Pizza for Breakfast*

Social Studies

Different countries specialize in different types of pizza. For example, the Neapolitan area of Italy uses sun-dried tomatoes and fish on their pizzas. Some German pizza includes liverwurst and ham. Research pizza from different countries or regions of one country. Make a bar graph to show the number of places that use similar ingredients. (MI = V/L, V/S, L/M)

Mathematics

Have you ever had a food that you could not finish? What did you do with the leftover food? After the whole class pizza party, determine a method for storing the leftover salad fixings or any leftover pizza. Use pint, quart, and gallon containers or plastic seal bags. Then help your parents divide your leftover food into refrigerator or freezer containers at home for a fun homework assignment. (MI = V/S, L/M)

Science

At times, life can be very busy and hectic. The main characters in the book were very busy and then they even got busier. Have you ever been so busy that you didn't have time to eat? That is very busy. Probably you may been so busy that you didn't have time to eat at home, but you resorted to eating fast food. In moderation, fast food can be a healthful choice. Fast food is always preferred over skipping a meal completely (unless there is a religious reason why you would skip a meal). Investigate why it's not healthy to skip meals. Usually fast food contains a high percentage of fat and salt, and the food selections are limited in fresh fruit and vegetables. Investigate the role of high fat and high sodium foods in the contribution of heart disease. (MI = I/I, V/L)

Language Arts

Like Frank and Zelda in the story, getting what you want does not always make you happy. Share a disappointment that you've had in your life with a classmate. After listening, write three sentences on how your friend could cope with the disappointment. Share your written ideas with one another. Choose one of the suggestions and write a reaction paragraph on how the idea might work for you. (MI = V/L, V/S, I/I, I/S)

Physical Education

Spinning pizza dough involves coordination and balance. Balance a paper plate on different parts of your body, e.g., head, elbow, knee, hand, and finger. Next spin a Frisbee on your finger and toss it into the air. Try to catch it. What body part besides your arm helps the Frisbee get into the air? (Skills developed: body part identification, dynamic balance, coordination). (MI = B/K)

Art

Bring an old or interestingly shaped bottle from home. Wrap these bottles with masking tape. Place a candle into the neck of the bottle to make a candle centerpiece for your class pizza party. Putty or clay may help to hold the candle in place until the wax from the burning candle drips onto the neck of the bottle. (MI = V/S)

Music

Invite a violin player from your local school or community orchestra to play during your class pizza party. Study the role of tempo in setting the mood of music. Why does a violin do this so well? (MI = M/R)

Across the Curriculum

Featured Book #3 of the Focused Theme: Diners, Restaurants, and Soup Kitchens	# Uncle Willie and the Soup Kitchen by DyAnne DiSalvo-Ryan Morrow Junior Books, 1991

This lesson addresses the following Dietary Guidelines for Americans:

⇒ *1. Eat a variety of foods.*
    2. Balance the food you eat with physical activity; maintain or improve your weight.
⇒ *3. Choose a diet with plenty of grain products, vegetables, and fruits.*
⇒ *4. Choose a diet low in fat, saturated fat, and cholesterol.*
    5. Choose a diet moderate in sugars.
    6. Choose a diet moderate in salt and sodium.
    7. Choose an alcohol and drug-free lifestyle.

This lesson highlights the following food groups from the Food Guide Pyramid:

⇒ *Bread, Cereal, Rice, & Pasta Group*
⇒ *Fruit Group*
⇒ *Vegetable Group*
⇒ *Milk, Yogurt, & Cheese Group*
⇒ *Meat, Poultry, Fish, Dry Beans, Eggs, & Nuts Group*

Food Guide Pyramid
A Guide to Daily Food Choices

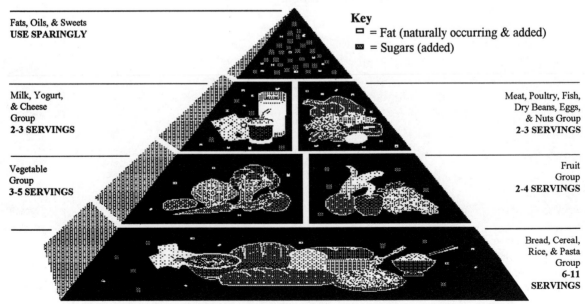

Source: U.S. Department of Agriculture & U.S. Department of Health and Human Services

130

Lesson Plans for Featured Book 3

DiSalvo-Ryan, D. (1991). <u>Uncle willie</u> and <u>the</u> <u>soup</u> <u>kitchen</u>. New York: Morrow Junior. A little boy has an Uncle Willie who works at a soup kitchen during the day. The little boy doesn't understand what a soup kitchen is so Uncle Willie takes him to work. They prepare and serve a meal to the poor people of the community. Advanced reading level.

Pre-Reading Activities for *Uncle Willie and the Soup Kitchen*

Can you think of situations where people have needed help? Describe a situation where you gave one or two people assistance. (MI = I/I, V/L)

Have you ever been really hungry? How did you feel when you were really hungry? How does hunger affect your feelings or mood? (MI = I/I, V/L)

Post-Reading Activities for *Uncle Willie and the Soup Kitchen*

Questions to develop thinking skills (Bloom's Taxonomy)

1. *Knowledge:*   What is Uncle Willie's job? Label his work responsibilities in a picture that you draw.

2. *Comprehension:*   Explain the various ways or reasons which bring people to eat at the soup kitchen.

3. *Application:*   Report the number of steps that the soup kitchen goes through in order to feed the people that come there.

4. *Analysis:*   Categorize the meal served at the soup kitchen into the five food groups. What food groups are not represented?

5. *Synthesis:*   Imagine the narrator's attitude toward the soup kitchen and the people that eat there. How does is it change as the story goes along?

6. *Evaluation:*   Consider the multiple ways in which a person can be healthy. In what ways are the people that visit the soup kitchen healthy?

Solo Work for *Uncle Willie and the Soup Kitchen*

In the story, the boy is somewhat afraid of the homeless people. He is also sad for the people because they are lonely. Uncle Willie is sad for the people but is not afraid. Uncle Willie has made friends with some of the people in his community. Review the story and find the phrases that support these observations. Make a list of activities or ideas that you can do to show you care for people. List the qualities of your closest friend. (MI = I/S, V/L)

Small Group Work for *Uncle Willie and the Soup Kitchen*

In groups of three or four, choose a soup recipe from a collection of cookbooks. Choose one recipe that is easy to make and requires no expensive or unusual ingredients; share your collection of recipes with your community soup kitchens. Carefully write out the recipes with the serving sizes included in the directions. Calculate how much of the ingredients would be needed to increase the recipe to 50 servings, 100 servings and 150 servings. (MI = L/M)

Whole Class Work for *Uncle Willie and the Soup Kitchen*

Ask a worker from a local soup kitchen or homeless shelter to talk to your class about the facility.
Before the guest speaker arrives, collect canned goods, art work, and paper products that could be used in the facility. You could also volunteer your gifts of labor to the facility. Ask the speaker if there are ways in which the class can help. Some examples might be helping to cut up vegetables for the kitchen or sorting canned goods in the pantry. Use the food guide pyramid at the end of this lesson plan which shows what foods are suitable for donation in food drives. (MI = I/S, B/K, V/L)

Across the Curriculum for
Uncle Willie and the Soup Kitchen
Social Studies

Discuss people or pets that have no place to live. Does homelessness effect their longevity? Does it effect their overall health? Does it effect how they bathe, eat, dress, sleep? Hunger is a terrible thing. Some people do not have enough money to buy food. Impoverished people can be at risk for nutritional diseases. When hunger occurs, blood glucose (sugar) drops. Food helps glucose to return to a normal level. When glucose is low, the mind cannot function properly. The person may be depressed and not able to work. Many just want to sleep or sit. A child who is constantly hungry cannot learn or take an exam. Have you ever been hungry? (MI = V/L)

Mathematics

Count the number of trash receptacles in the story. Count the number in your classroom, in your home, or on a walk in your community. Compare your results by making a class bar graph. Discuss the virtues of cleanliness and the importance of not littering. Many objects and materials can be recycled for money. What materials does your community recycle? On a class cleanup day, collect these materials and turn them in for cash. Donate your money to a local charity. How much money did you make as a class? Divide the time you spent with the number of individuals who worked. How much did you each earn per hour? (MI = M/L, I/S)

Science

Investigate the cooling time of soup in a bowl and a cup. Measure the temperature of the soup in each container at five-minute intervals. Which cools faster? Does the number of vegetables and grains in the soup make a difference? Does the material that the bowl and cup are made of make a difference? (MI = B/K, L/M)

Language Arts

Read the author's notes in the book called "About Soup Kitchens". Write a letter on behalf of the homeless people or animals. This could be an advocacy letter written by yourself or as a class. Maybe send your letters by electronic mail to state or federal officials. Share your letters with your principal before mailing them. Also send your letter to your local newspaper. (MI = I/I, V/L)

Physical Education

Play trash can basketball like shown in the book. (MI = B/K, L/M)

Art

Make colored-pencil drawings as shown in the book. Take your artwork to a local soup kitchen or food pantry to be displayed. The method for making illustrations in the book is found on the copyright page. Invite a local artist or your school art teacher to explain the statement, i.e., "The text is 13 point ITC Cushing Book". (MI = V/S)

Music

Create a "Shoe String Band" by using toilet paper-roll kazoos, boxes, pot lids for cymbals, cookie cans for drums, and spoons on the knee. What fun! (MI = B/K, M/R)

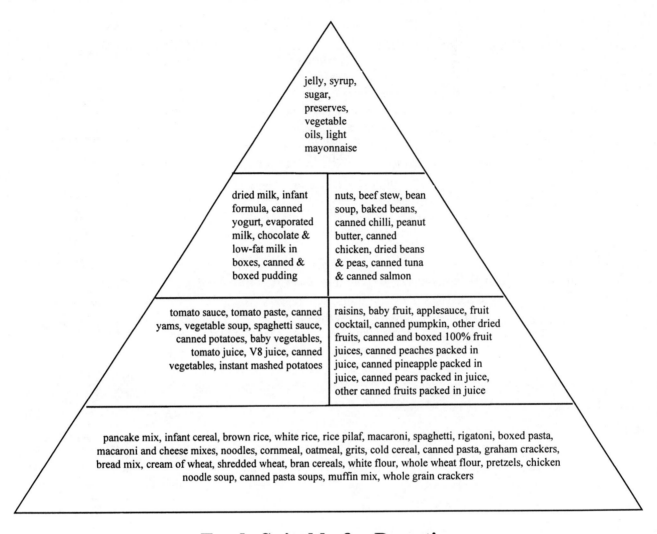

**Foods Suitable for Donation
in Food Drives**

Source: Krummel, D.A. (1994). National nutrition month and hunger awareness week: A win-win effort. *Journal of the American Dietetic Association, 94(3)*, 254-255.

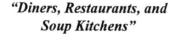
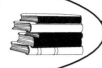

Other Books to Read for
"Diners, Restaurants, and Soup Kitchens"

This list contains excellent books to read for learning about Diners, Restaurants, and Soup Kitchens. Use these books along with the Featured Books when teaching the lessons on the previous pages.

Florian, D. (1992). A chef. New York: Greenwillow Books.
> The life of a chef is a busy one! A chef starts her day off at the market, buys and cleans the food, then prepares it. Finally, the restaurant opens and the hungry customers are served.

Gibbons, G. (1989). Marge's diner. New York: HarperCollins Children's Books.
> Everyone goes to Marge's Diner because it is open 24 hours a day. Marge feeds all kinds of people: truckdrivers, families, travelers, school kids, businessmen, and telephone company workers. Everyone is friendly at the diner, and it is a big meeting place for friends.

Kroll, S. (1991). Howard and gracie's luncheonette. New York: Henry Holt & Co., Inc.
> Howard and Gracie own a "luncheonette". They describe the work that they do and all the people that come to eat there.

Viorst, J. (1992). The good-bye book. New York: Macmillan Children's Book Group.
> A boy doesn't want his parents to go to a restaurant and leave him with a sitter. He begs and pleads with them and won't say good-bye. When he realizes the sitter is nice, he says good-bye.

Letter to Food Service Professionals

Our class is starting on a new learning adventure called "Let's Make a Meal". We will learn about *when* we eat (first graders), *where* we eat and buy food (second graders), and *with whom* we eat and enjoy food (third graders). Since Food Service Professionals are responsible for coordinating and offering the School Breakfast Program and School Lunch Program, we would like to invite you to our class to learn more about the foods you offer us. Is our school a participant in these federally funded programs? We think it is fun that we can eat at the school cafeteria. Is our cafeteria a type of diner? Is it a restaurant? Is it a soup kitchen? Why or why not? Why do some schools have fast food restaurants in their cafeterias? Who buys all the food for our school? Does one person go to the grocery store or market to buy all the food? What bakeries or vendors come to our cafeteria to deliver food or beverages? Where does leftover food go after the meal? How many workers are there in the cafeteria? What do they do behind the scenes before and after a meal? Who is the designated chef or lead cook for our school? Has that person ever worked in a diner, restaurant, or soup kitchen? Do the same people work during the School Breakfast Program and the School Lunch Program? What is meant by shift work? Why don't we tip the cafeteria workers like we tip waiters and waitresses at a sit-down restaurant?

You can tell that we are very eager to learn about how meals are made, served, and coordinated at our school on a daily basis. We have many, many more questions to ask you and your staff too. Thank you for helping us learn more about your job. Please feel free to visit our classroom this month as we explore the exciting topic of meals!

Thank you for helping us to learn!

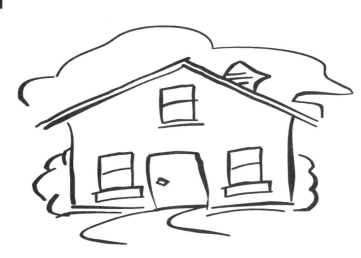

Letter to Parents and Caregivers

We are starting another nutrition and health unit called "Let's Make a Meal". We will learn about *when* we eat (first graders), *where* we eat and buy food (second graders), and *with whom* we eat and enjoy food (third graders). In order for this to be a meaningful learning experience for our class, would you please contribute one of the needed items below? Anything you can do to help us by _____ (date) will be greatly appreciated. We will also appreciate your assistance during some of our classroom and community lessons in this unit.

- 1 skeen yarn or heavy string
- 1 box or bag of uncooked pasta
- A favorite pancake recipe, including the ingredients to make one batch of the pancakes
- 1 box of prepared pancake mix
- Used metal, cloth, or vinyl lunch boxes
- Paper lunch bags
- 1 package of balloons
- Empty and clean food cartons, containers, or boxes
- 1 jug or bottle of syrup for pancakes
- Toppings for pancakes
- Old buttons, spangles, or glittery decorations
- One yard of cloth
- Use of a video camera and tape
- 1 package of vegetables _____
- 1 package of straws
- 10 feet of butcher paper
- 1 bag of oranges or apples
- 1 can of_____ soup
- 1 package of shaped pretzels
- 1 cup of flour, sugar or 1 package of yeast

Thank you kindly!

For the Pleasure of Reading

This booklist can be sent home during Unit 3: Let's Make a Meal, so that your students and their families can read additional literature about food and nutrition together. You can also place these books in your classroom library during the unit. These books are considered secondary resources for this unit. Each book and its abstract is listed as a primary resource in another unit. Use the index at the back of this book to see how titles are crosslisted with other units. Our goal is to show how each book can be used in multiple ways to teach nutrition and health concepts.

Breakfast, Lunch, and Dinner

Adams, J. (1991). Going for oysters. Morton Grove, IL: Albert Whitman & Company.

Baron-Hall, D. (1989). Only at the children's table. Chathem, NJ: Raintree Steck-Vaughn.

Brown, M. (1951). Skipper john's cook. New York: Charles Scribner's Sons.

Choi, S. N. (1993). Halmoni and the picnic. Boston: Houghton Mifflin Co.

de Regniers, B. S. (1989). May i bring a friend? New York: McClelland & Stewart Ltd.

dePaola, T. (1974). Watch out for the chicken feet in your soup. New York: Simon & Schuster.

DiSalvo-Ryan, D. (1991). Uncle willie and the soup kitchen. New York: Morrow Junior Books.

Drucker, M. (1992). Grandma's latkes. San Diego: Harcourt Brace & Co.

Falwell, C. (1993). Feast for 10. New York: Scholastic Inc.

Feder, P. K. (1992). Where does the teacher live? New York: Dutton Children's Books.

Freidman, I. R. (1984). How my parents learned to eat. Boston: Houghton Mifflin Co.

Hudson, W. (1993). I love my family. New York: Scholastic Inc.

Kroll, S. (1991). Howard and gracie's luncheonette. New York: Henry Holt & Co., Inc.

Manushkin, F. (1995). The matzah that papa brought home. New York: Scholastic Inc.

Mitchell, B., & Sandford, J. (1993). Down buttermilk lane. New York: Lothrop, Lee & Shepard.

Nerlove, M. (1989). Passover. Niles, IL: Albert Whitman & Company.

Nikola-Lisa, W. (1991). 1,2,3 thanksgiving. Morton Grove, IL: Albert Whitman & Company.

Otey, M. (1993). Blue moon soup spoon. New York: Farrar, Straus & Giroux.

Polacco, P. (1988). Rechenka's eggs. New York: Philomel Books.

Rattigan, J. K. (1993). Dumpling soup. New York: Little, Brown & Co.

Rice, E. (1990). At grammy's house. New York: Greenwillow Books.

Saunders, S. (1982). Fish fry. New York: Puffin Books.

Soto, G., & Martinez, E. (1993). Too many tamales. New York: Putnam Publishing Group.

Steffy, J. (1987). The school picnic. Intercourse, PA: Good Books.

Tobias, T. (1993). Pot luck. New York: Lothrop, Lee and Shepard Books.

Weston, M. (1994). Apple juice tea. New York: Houghton Mifflin Company.

Williams, J. (1992). Playtime 123. New York: Dial Books For Young Readers.

Wood, A. (1987). Heckedy peg. San Diego: Scholastic Inc.

For the Pleasure of Reading, cont'd

Markets, Bakeries, and Vendors
Aliki. (1979). <u>The two of them</u>. New York: William Morrow & Co., Inc.
Bider, D. (1989). <u>A drop of honey</u>. New York: Simon & Schuster Books for Young Readers.
Darling, B. (1992). <u>Valerie and the silver pear</u>. New York: Macmillan Children's Book Group.
dePaola, T. (1993). <u>Tom</u>. New York: Scholastic Inc.
dePaola, T. (1989). <u>Tony's bread</u>. New York: Putnam Publishing Group.
DiSalvo-Ryan, D. (1991). <u>Uncle willie and the soup kitchen</u>. New York: Morrow Junior Books.
Florian, D. (1992). <u>A chef</u>. New York: Greenwillow Books.
Goldin, B. D. (1993). <u>Cakes and miracles: A purim tale</u>. New York: Puffin Books.
Hines, A. G. (1988). <u>Daddy makes the best spaghetti</u>. New York: Houghton Mifflin Co.
Jaspersohn, W. (1993). <u>Cookies</u>. New York: Macmillan Children's Book Group.
Kelley, T. (1989). <u>Let's eat</u>. New York: Dutton Children's Books.
Kroll, S. (1989). <u>The hokey-pokey man</u>. New York: Holiday House Inc.
McDonald, M. (1994). <u>The potato man</u>. New York: Orchard Books.
Mitchell, B., & Sandford, J. (1993). <u>Down buttermilk lane</u>. New York: Lothrop, Lee and Shepard.
Olaleye, I. (1994). <u>Bitter bananas</u>. Honesdale, PA: Boyd's Mill Press.
Spurr, E. (1991). <u>The biggest birthday cake in the world</u>. San Diego: Harcourt Brace & Co.
Tobias, T. (1993). <u>Pot luck</u>. New York: Lothrop, Lee and Shepard Books.
Valens, A. (1993). <u>Danilo the fruitman</u>. New York: Dial Books For Young Readers.
Watson, P., & Watson, M. (1994). <u>The market lady and the mango tree</u>. New York: Wm. Morrow.

Diners, Restaurants, and Soup Kitchens
Freidman, I. R. (1984). <u>How my parents learned to eat</u>. Boston: Houghton Mifflin Co.
Howard, E. F. (1991). <u>Aunt flossie's hat (and crab cakes later)</u>. New York: Dell Publishers Co, Inc.
Kelley, T. (1989). <u>Let's eat</u>. New York: Dutton Children's Books.

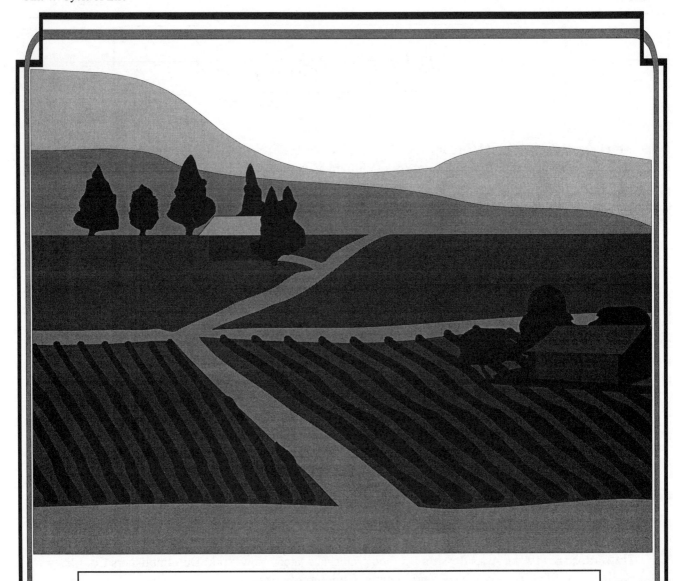

Unit 4:
<u>Cycle of Life</u>

Down on the Farm

Unit 4: Cycle of Life

Instructional activities for Unit 4 have been designed to achieve the *National Health Education Standards.* The performances that students will know and do for this unit are listed below each standard.

⟹ 1. **Students will comprehend concepts related to health promotion and disease prevention.**
Performance Indicators. As a result of health instruction in Grades K-4, students will
  4. Describe how the family influences personal health.
  5. Describe how physical, social, and emotional environments influence personal health.
  6. Identify health problems that should be detected and treated early.

⟹ 2. **Students will demonstrate the ability to access valid health information and health-promotion products and services.**
Performance Indicators. As a result of health instruction in Grades K-4, students will
  1. Identify characteristics of valid health information and health-promoting products & services.
  2. Demonstrate the ability to locate resources from home, school, and community that provide valid health information.
  3. Explain how media influences the selection of health information, products, & services.

⟹ 3. **Students will demonstrate the ability to practice health-enhancing behaviors and reduce health risks.**
Performance Indicators. As a result of health instruction in Grades K-4, students will
  1. Identify responsible health behaviors.
  3. Compare behaviors that are safe to those that are risky or harmful.
  5. Develop injury prevention and management strategies for personal health.

⟹ 4. **Students will analyze the influence of culture, media, technology, and other factors on health.**
Performance Indicators. As a result of health instruction in Grades K-4, students will
  1. Describe how culture influences personal health behaviors.
  2. Explain how media influences thoughts, feelings, and health behaviors.
  3. Describe ways technology can influence personal health.

⟹ 5. **Students will demonstrate the ability to use interpersonal communication skills to enhance health.**
Performance Indicators. As a result of health instruction in Grades K-4, students will
  2. describe characteristics needed to be a responsible friend and family member.
  5. demonstrate attentive listening skills to build and maintain healthy relationships.
  8. demonstrate non-violent strategies to resolve conflicts.

⟹ 6. **Students will demonstrate the ability to use goal setting and decision-making skills to enhance health.**
Performance Indicators. As a result of health instruction in Grades K-4, students will
  2. explain when to ask for assistance in making health-related decisions and setting health goals.

⟹ 7. **Students will demonstrate the ability to advocate for personal, family, & community health.**
Performance Indicators. As a result of health instruction in Grades K-4, students will
  3. identify community agencies that advocate for healthy individuals, families, and communitities.

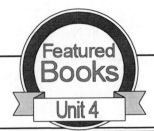

Overall Featured Book for Unit 4

Locker, T. (1994). Family farm. New York: Puffin Books.
    Mike tells the story about the life and hardships of living on a farm. Because of many factors, they decide to start selling pumpkins and flowers which enable them to remain on the farm. Intermediate reading level.

Books for Focused Theme: Down on the Farm

Gibbons, G. (1988). Farming. New York: Holiday House Inc.
    Farms are filled with exciting things! There are animals being born, crops being planted then harvested, and cleaning being done. During each season, there are different chores to do on the farm. Intermediate reading level.

Paulsen, G. (1995). The tortilla factory. San Diego: Harcourt Brace and Co.
    In the spring, a tiny yellow corn seed is planted. From that corn seed, a tortilla shell is created. The tortilla shell gives strength to the workers. The entire process will be repeated the following spring. Intermediate reading level.

Slawson, M. B. (1994). Apple picking time. New York: Crown Publishers.
    A little girl goes with her family to pick apples at harvest time. After picking a long time, she finally fills her whole bin and gets a mark on a ticket that she accomplished her goal. Advanced reading level.

| Unit 4: Cycle of Life
Scope & Sequence of Nutrition Content | | | | Grade 2 |

Nutrition Content: Dietary Guidelines	*Family Farm*	*Farming*	*The Tortilla Factory*	*Apple Picking Time*
Eat a variety of foods		X		
Balance food with exercise	X	X	X	X
Choose grains, vegetables, and fruits	X	X	X	X
Choose low fat and low cholesterol				
Choose moderate sugars		X		
Choose moderate salt and sodium				

Nutrition Content: Food Groups	*Family Farm*	*Farming*	*The Tortilla Factory*	*Apple Picking Time*
Bread, Cereal, Rice, & Pasta Group		X	X	
Fruit Group		X		X
Vegetable Group	X	X	X	
Milk, Yogurt, & Cheese Group	X	X		
Meat, Poultry, Fish, Dry Beans, Eggs, & Nuts Group		X		
Fats, Oils, & Sweets Group				

<table>
<tr><td>

Overall Featured Book
of
Unit 4: Cycle of Life

</td><td>

Family Farm
by Thomas Locker
Puffin Books, 1994

</td></tr>
</table>

This lesson addresses the following Dietary Guidelines for Americans:

1. Eat a variety of foods.
⇒ *2. Balance the food you eat with physical activity; maintain or improve your weight.*
⇒ *3. Choose a diet with plenty of grain products, vegetables, and fruits.*
4. Choose a diet low in fat, saturated fat, and cholesterol.
5. Choose a diet moderate in sugars.
6. Choose a diet moderate in salt and sodium.
7. Choose an alcohol and drug-free lifestyle.

This lesson highlights the following food groups from the Food Guide Pyramid:

Bread, Cereal, Rice, & Pasta Group
Fruit Group
⇒ *Vegetable Group*
⇒ *Milk, Yogurt, & Cheese Group*
Meat, Poultry, Fish, Dry Beans, Eggs, & Nuts Group

Food Guide Pyramid
A Guide to Daily Food Choices

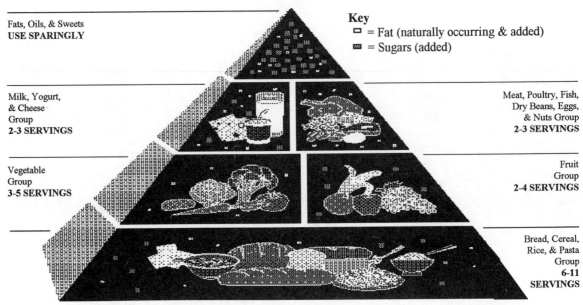

Source: U.S. Department of Agriculture & U.S. Department of Health and Human Services

Lesson Plans for Overall Featured Book

Locker, T. (1994). <u>Family</u> <u>farm</u>. New York: Puffin Books.
Mike tells the story about the life and hardships of living on a farm. Because of many factors, they decide to start selling pumpkins and flowers which enable them to remain on the farm. Intermediate reading level.

Pre-Reading Activities for *Family Farm*

Visit a farm or a petting zoo. (MI = B/K)

Invite a cooperative extension (4-H) agent into your classroom for a visit. Discuss the role of program participants in showing food, animals, plants, clothing, and crafts at the state fair. (MI = V/L)

Contact your local Farm Bureau agent for a classroom visit. Since this book, *Family Farm*, won the Ohio Farm Bureau Women's Award for Children's Literature, perhaps a member of your local bureau would like to read it to the class. Does your state have a children's literature award for farming-related storylines? (MI = V/L)

Post-Reading Activities for *Family Farm*

Questions to develop thinking skills (Bloom's Taxonomy)

1. Knowledge: Name the people who live on this farm.

2. Comprehension: Restate the problem that Sarah and Mike faced. How did they decide to help?

3. Application: Role play the conversation the family had around the dinner table. Role play the conversation with different feelings.

4. Analysis: Categorize the chores and activities that Sarah and Mike did before school and after school.

5. Synthesis: Imagine the feelings of all the family members if the family had to move to the city. How might their attitudes towards each other change?

6. Evaluation: Judge the family's decision to 'stick it out'. Do you think the decisions they made were good ones? What qualities of this family do these decisions show?

Solo Work for *Family Farm*

Write a story about a visit to a farm or county fair. Illustrate your story with artwork or pictures cut out of magazines or a newspaper. (MI = V/L, V/S)

Small Group Work for *Family Farm*

Form small teams of two or three to investigate current prices of local crops and animal products. Each team could investigate one or more items, then report to the whole class for a whole class project. Student-generated questions are encouraged. Some suggested teacher-generated questions might be as follows:

Listen to the farm reports on the local radio and read farm prices in the local newspaper.
How often do these prices change? Who determines these prices?

Do you know how these farm commodities are used in your school breakfast and school lunch? Ask your Food Service Professional in your school to talk about these commodities. What prices were the commodities in the book worth?

Investigate the price of seeds, water, land, and chemicals needed to raise these crops or to keep the animals healthy. How much would the farmer have to earn on his crops or milk to be able to keep the farm? (MI = V/L, L/M, I/S)

Whole Class Work for *Family Farm*

Invite a member of your local chapter of the National Dairy Council to come to class. Ask them to bring educational materials like pamplets, games, and videos to class. Have students also arrange for a local farmer to visit the classroom to talk about family life on the farm.

On the day of the guest speaker, hold a Tasting Festival for different types of milk (e.g., whole milk, 1/2%, 1%, 2%, skim milk, chocolate milk, reconstituted dried milk, sweetened condensed milk) or cheeses. Discuss the amount of fat found in whole milk (3.5%), 2%, and skim milk (<1%). Mozzerella cheese has less fat than other white or yellow cheeses. Compare fat grams in cheeses made with partially skimmed milk. Compare nutrient content and taste of cream cheeses that are low in fat, have no fat, and regular (5% fat). (MI = V/L, B/K, L/M)

Across the Curriculum for *Family Farm*

Social Studies

Compare families that live on farms and families that live in non-rural communities. Compare different types of farm families. For example, dairy farms, hog farms, crop farms, combination livestock and crop farms, and ranches. (MI = V/L)

Mathematics

Investigate the current price of crops and animal products in your area. Is this price increasing or decreasing? Compare with last year at this time. Make up math word problems, for example, if you have 100 acres of corn and each acre gives 80 bushes of corn. A bushel if worth two dollars, what is the corn value of the 100 acres? (MI = L/M)

Science

Plant bean seeds in a jar and place in the dark. No soil is required but water is needed. Check every three days. Bean seeds will become bean sprouts in about a week. Cook and enjoy or eat raw. (MI = B/K)

Language Arts

Name different farm animals, their offspring, and what foods they produce or become. For example, cows make milk which can become cheese and butter. Cattle or steer become steak and roasts. Baby calves can become... (MI = V/L)

Physical Education

When weeding a garden, farmers can either use a hoe or a large tractor with a cultivator. What method requires more physical activity? Using a hoe for a long period of time can create lower back strain and pain. How can you stretch your lower back and strengthen your abdomen, so your lower back can withstand the stress of bending over a hoe? (Skills: Sit cross legged and lean forward to place your elbows and forearms on the floor. Pause for five seconds to stretch your lower back. Next lay on your back with your arms crossed in front of your chest and your knees bent. Curl your shoulders and head toward your knees then return to your back. Repeat as many times as you can several times per week.) (MI = B/K)

Art

Make a poster for your cafeteria which shows how a food or animal product is used for food. Coordinate the display of your posters with the food menu for the week. (MI = V/S)

Music

Play the Raffi song "Down on Grandpa's Farm" (See Teaching Resources in the back of the book). Make up a routine of dancing and marching and pantomime to the song as you sing it. (MI = M/R, B/K)

Across the Curriculum

Focused Theme: Down on the Farm

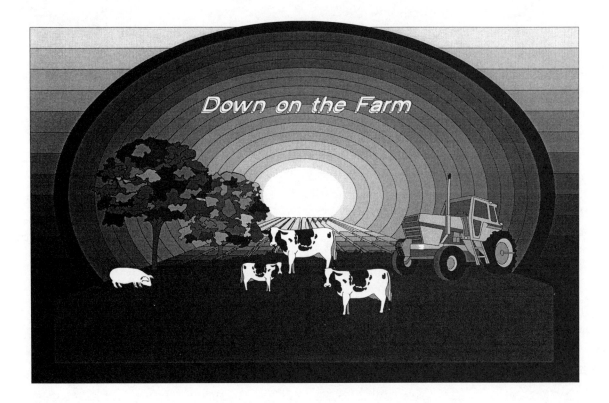

Down on the Farm

<u>Overview of Down on the Farm:</u>

This focused theme looks at where plant foods are grown and harvested and where animal products are produced and marketed. This section also highlights the cycle of life on a farm for plants and animals. Some historical and cultural backgrounds of food are investigated. Since farm life requires hard work, the social and economic aspects of living and working on a farm are explored through several of the featured books.

Featured Book #1
of the Focused Theme:
Down on the Farm

Farming
by Gail Gibbons
Holiday House, 1988

This lesson addresses the following Dietary Guidelines for Americans:
⇒   *1. Eat a variety of foods.*
⇒   *2. Balance the food you eat with physical activity; maintain or improve your weight.*
⇒   *3. Choose a diet with plenty of grain products, vegetables, and fruits.*
        4. Choose a diet low in fat, saturated fat, and cholesterol.
⇒   *5. Choose a diet moderate in sugars.*
        6. Choose a diet moderate in salt and sodium.
        7. Choose an alcohol and drug-free lifestyle.

This lesson highlights the following food groups from the Food Guide Pyramid:
⇒   *Bread, Cereal, Rice, & Pasta Group*
⇒   *Fruit Group*
⇒   *Vegetable Group*
⇒   *Milk, Yogurt, & Cheese Group*
⇒   *Meat, Poultry, Fish, Dry Beans, Eggs, & Nuts Group*

Food Guide Pyramid
A Guide to Daily Food Choices

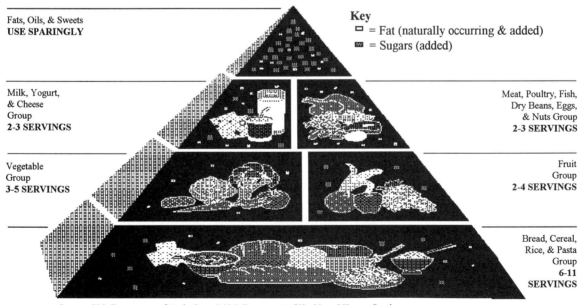

Source: U.S. Department of Agriculture & U.S. Department of Health and Human Services

Lesson Plans for Featured Book 1

Gibbons, G. (1988). <u>Farming</u>. New York: Holiday House Inc.
Farms are filled with exciting things! There are animals being born, crops being planted then harvested, and cleaning being done. During each season, there are different chores to do on the farm. Intermediate reading level.

Pre-Reading Activities for *Farming*

Look at a calendar to chart the planting and harvesting schedule of local crops in your area. (MI = L/M)

Visit a farm equipment store to compare different tractors, cultivators, disks, bailers, harvesters, and dusters. (MI = B/K)

Post-Reading Activities for *Farming*

<u>Questions to develop thinking skills</u> (Bloom's Taxonomy)

1. Knowledge: Name the inside chores in the summer that were shown in *Farming*.

2. Comprehension: Review the various types of farms. Is there a farm for each of the five food groups? What are they?

3. Application: Put in order the steps to grow vegetables.

4. Analysis: Compare four seasons on the farm. Observe the changes in each of the seasons. How do events and chores change and why?

5. Synthesis: Create a new type of machine which will make harvesting a fruit or vegetable easier.

6. Evaluation: Decide whether or not you would like to live or work on a farm? Why or why not?

Solo Work for *Farming*

Draw a vegetable garden that you would like to plant. Name and label the plants. Look at the food guide pyramid to see examples of vegetables. Each student can place soil into a paper cup, then plant a vegetable seed. Place all of the seed cups into a tray of water and in the sun at a classroom window. As a whole class project, the seeds can be transplanted into a garden plot at your school or could be taken home for family gardens. Potatoes and yams may be placed in a cup of water and fixed in place with toothpicks so they grow long roots. Alfalfa seeds may be planted on a sponge or wet toweling, then placed in the sun light and kept moist for growth. (MI = V/S, B/K, V/L)

Small Group Work for *Farming*

Organize your class into small groups of two or three for a Food Tasting of Fresh Vegetables. (MI = I/S, B/K, V/L)

Teachers should:
- Obtain washed vegetables such as celery, carrots, broccoli, cauliflower, red and green peppers, jicama, oriental peas, radishes, and zucchini.
- Buy or make a low-fat dip for the vegetables. Also buy individual dipping cups for use by each student to reduce the spreading of germs.
- Obtain small paper plates, napkins, and small paper cups for the food tasting.
- Invite parents, local grocer, or food service professional to assist with the food tasting.
- Fix work stations with trays, cutting boards, and round-tipped knives.
- Organize and supervise small groups of students to cut and arrange a variety of vegetables on each vegetable tray. Discuss how to make the trays of vegetables visually appealing.
- Suggest that students try at least four different vegetables. Help students decide which vegetables they would award 1st, 2nd, and 3rd choice ribbons.

Students should:
- Wash hands with soap and warm running water as modeled by the teacher.
- On a cutting board, carefully cut or separate vegetables into bite-sized pieces.
- Arrange a variety of vegetables on each tray. Alternate different colors of vegetables on the trays for appeal. Place toothpicks into some of the vegetables for ease in picking up.
- Set each place at the table with a plate, napkin, vegetable dip cup, and drinking cup. Water, milk, or vegetable juice could be served.
- Eat at least four different vegetables. Decide which vegetables receive your 1st, 2nd, and 3rd choice for taste.
- Write several sentences to describe your first choice vegetable. Describe your vegetable in color, shape, smell, taste, and texture.

Whole Class Work for *Farming*

Take a class vote on the 1st, 2nd, and 3rd choice vegetables. In cooperative learning teams, research the history and nutrient value of the top three vegetables. Additional vegetables can be researched for more variety. Reports can be shared with the entire class. Encourage fact sheets, posters, songs, and skits to present the material. (MI = L/M, I/S, V/L, B/K, M/R)

Across the Curriculum for *Farming*

Social Studies

Study the way that farms have become mechanized over the past fifty years. Make two timelines to show how food production from animals and plants are similar and different from the increases in technology. (MI = V/S, L/M)

Mathematics

Brainstorm the many chores that need to be done on a farm during the spring, summer, fall and winter months. Next make a chart with each student's name and a list of chores for one season. Mark which chores each student would be willing to do during the selected season. Repeat the process for another season or two. Have each student rank order their seasonal preferences for working on a farm. (MI = V/L, I/S)

Science

What is the technology that preserves the nutrients in the food? Some examples are canning, freezing, and drying of foods. The oldest method was to dry foods in the sun or place them in a warm oven or over a fire. Drying removed the moisture from the food. Pioneers used spring houses or ice houses to help extend the shelf life of the food. A scientist, Jean Apparette, placed food in champagne bottles (because they are very heavy glass) to boil it for several hours. This preserved the food. Today we know this method as canning. Research the newest method of food preservation called irradiation. Visit the grocery store to look for irradiated food. (MI = V/L, B/K)

Language Arts

Discuss the health issues of farming. For example, what are the effects of excessive sun on your skin, lung exposure to fertilizers and insecticides, or lack of sleep due to heavy work loads? Select one of these issues as a class. Each student should contribute at least 5 sentences to a class book on the topic. Obtain brochures and pamphlets from your local American Cancer Society, American Lung Association, or Cooperative Extension to help you understand the issue. (MI = V/L)

Physical Education

Create a "people" farm machine. Divide your class into groups of eight to ten students. One student moves a body part and makes a noise "in place". A second child adds to the machine by moving in a different way. Continue until a group machine is in complete motion. This activity builds cooperation, creativity, and non-locomotor movements. (MI = I/S, B/K)

Art

Using small, medium, and large cardboard boxes, design a farm implement that helps to harvest food crops. Be sure to include safety devices or switches to the creations. (MI = V/S)

Music

During a quiet time or lunch time, play the Raffi song called "Naturally" (See the Teaching Resource in the back of the book). You can also combine sounds and rhythms to the people farm machine you make under Physical Education on this page. (MI = M/R)

Across the Curriculum

*Featured Book #2
of the Focused Theme:
Down on the Farm*

The Tortilla Factory
by Gary Paulsen
Harcourt Brace & Company, 1995

This lesson addresses the following Dietary Guidelines for Americans:

1. Eat a variety of foods.
⇒ 2. *Balance the food you eat with physical activity; maintain or improve your weight.*
⇒ 3. *Choose a diet with plenty of grain products, vegetables, and fruits.*
4. Choose a diet low in fat, saturated fat, and cholesterol.
5. Choose a diet moderate in sugars.
6. Choose a diet moderate in salt and sodium.
7. Choose an alcohol and drug-free lifestyle.

This lesson highlights the following food groups from the Food Guide Pyramid:

⇒ *Bread, Cereal, Rice, & Pasta Group*
Fruit Group
⇒ *Vegetable Group*
Milk, Yogurt, & Cheese Group
Meat, Poultry, Fish, Dry Beans, Eggs, & Nuts Group

Food Guide Pyramid
A Guide to Daily Food Choices

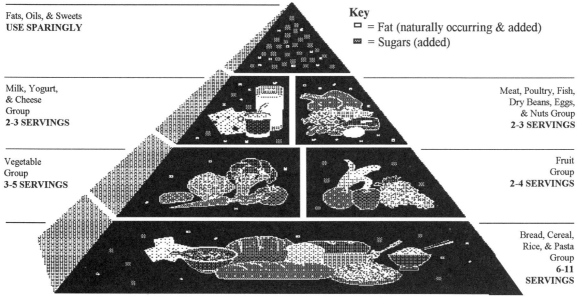

Source: U.S. Department of Agriculture & U.S. Department of Health and Human Services

Lesson Plans for Featured Book 2

Paulsen, G. (1995). <u>The <u>tortilla</u> <u>factory</u>. San Diego: Harcourt Brace and Co.
In the spring, a tiny yellow corn seed is planted. From that corn seed, a tortilla
shell is created. The tortilla shell gives strength to the workers. The entire
process will be repeated the following spring. Intermediate reading level.

Pre-Reading Activities for *The Tortilla Factory*

Ask students if they have ever planted crops or flowers. Discuss the cycle of life of plants. What is
their favorite part of the life cycle? (MI = V/L)

Ask students to describe a tortilla. What country originally made tortillas? How many different ways
have you eaten tortillas? (MI = V/L)

Post-Reading Activities for *The Tortilla Factory*

<u>Questions to develop thinking skills</u> (Bloom's Taxonomy)

1. Knowledge: Tell where corn goes after it is picked off the stalk.

2. Comprehension: Retell the story about the corn from the farm to the table. Explain the
role of the farmer in this cycle of life.

3. Application: Report on the uses for the corn other than to make tortillas.

4. Analysis: Think of another food that has a similar cycle of life. Compare this to corn.

5. Synthesis: Write a list of fillings for a tortilla using a food from each of the five food groups.

6. Evaluation: Choose a different corn product to eat for breakfast, lunch, and dinner.
Recommend one of the foods to a friend or family member based upon
the least amount of time for preparing it.

Solo Work for *The Tortilla Factory*

Design a tortilla or nacho. Draw and color your food and the ingredients, then cut and paste them onto another piece of paper. List the ingredients that you selected for your tortilla or nachos. What categories of the food pyramid does your tortilla or nachos contain? Compare your ingredient list with a restaurant brochure which lists the nutrient and caloric value of its foods. Ingredient lists are available free of charge from fast-food restaurants. (MI = V/S, L/M)

Small Group Work for *The Tortilla Factory*

Place 3 to 5 students into small groups to make a tortilla or nacho. Make a recipe card for the ingredients for the tortilla or nachos, then make a grocery list of the ingredients. Calculate how many ingredients are needed so that every person will get a bite-sized piece. Compare the cost of buying the ingredients in bulk with the cost of buying the food at a restaurant. (MI = I/S, V/L, V/S, L/M)

Whole Class Work *The Tortilla Factory*

Each small group will prepare their food for the class. When all foods are prepared, each group will explain the selected ingredients of their tortilla or nachos by writing them on the board. Foods will be served buffet style to the class. One student from each group will serve the food. Using a thumbs up or thumb down technique, students will vote on the different foods served that day. Compile a class recipe booklet for tortillas and nachos. Showcase the recipe booklets in the cafeteria during the week that similar foods are made by the food service professionals. Send the recipes home for parents and guardians to try. Encourage students to help prepare the meal at home. (MI = V/L, B/K, V/S, L/M)

Across the Curriculum for *The Tortilla Factory*

Social Studies

Investigate the role that corn played in the Native American culture or how this new world food changed the world. How many varieties of corn are there? Some examples are blue maize, popcorn, field corn, Indian corn, and strawberry corn. The kernels of corn in early American life were of many different colors on a much smaller corn cob. A descendant of Indian corn is sold today during autumn. Make a list of foods that are made of corn. Some examples are popcorn, cornflakes, cornbread, and corn tortilla. Today corn is grown for animal food and for human food. People use corn as corn on the cob, breading on fish, hush puppies, and corn bread. How many other ways do you eat corn? What would a movie be without popcorn? The term "hush puppies" has a very interesting history. When the pioneers would catch fish and fry it for dinner, their dogs would beg for pieces of fish to eat. The cook would take a small piece of cornbread mixture and fry it in the same skillet as the fish. When the cornbread was done, the cook would give it to the dogs and say "Eat this and hush puppies". Today hush puppies are served with fish in certain parts of the country. Mmm! Good. (MI = V/L)

Mathematics

Count the numbers of rows on an ear of corn. Do all ears of corn have the same number of rows? Graph or chart your findings. (MI = V/S, L/M)

Science

Investigate the pollination of corn. Compare the roles of female and male plants. How long is the growing period for corn? Compare corn varieties in seed catalogs. Write a paragraph comparing the differences between two different varieties of corn. (MI = V/L)

Language Arts

Describe how you eat corn on the cob. Do you eat across or around the ear? Do you eat from the small end or the big end? Do you put anything on your corn? What other unique aspects of corn eating can you describe? After you verbalize your answers with a classmate, put your responses in writing. (MI = B/K, V/L, I/S)

Physical Education

Mixing tortilla dough requires strong arms and hands. List three sport activities that require strong arm muscles. How could you develop arm or hand strength for one of the sports? Squeeze a tennis ball in your hand five times. How do the muscles in your forearms feel? Skills developed include forearm strength and endurance. (MI = B/K)

Art

Make corn shuck dolls or animals. Place the corn shucks in water until tender. Design the shape of the doll or animal, let it dry, then decorate. (MI = B/K, V/S)

Music

Play the Raffi song called "Nations" (See the Teaching Resources in the back of the book). Listen to the names of the different Native American tribes. Beat drums and shake rattles at the beginning and at the end of the song. Which of these Native American tribes had festivals and dances to honor corn as a food? (MI = M/R, V/L)

Across the Curriculum

*Featured Book #3
of the Focused Theme:
Down on the Farm*

Apple Picking Time
by Michele Benoit Slawson
Crown Publishers, Inc., 1994

This lesson addresses the following Dietary Guidelines for Americans:

1. Eat a variety of foods.
⇒ *2. Balance the food you eat with physical activity; maintain or improve your weight.*
⇒ *3. Choose a diet with plenty of grain products, vegetables, and fruits.*
4. Choose a diet low in fat, saturated fat, and cholesterol.
5. Choose a diet moderate in sugars.
6. Choose a diet moderate in salt and sodium.
7. Choose an alcohol and drug-free lifestyle.

This lesson highlights the following food groups from the Food Guide Pyramid:

Bread, Cereal, Rice, & Pasta Group
⇒ *Fruit Group*
Vegetable Group
Milk, Yogurt, & Cheese Group
Meat, Poultry, Fish, Dry Beans, Eggs, & Nuts Group

Food Guide Pyramid
A Guide to Daily Food Choices

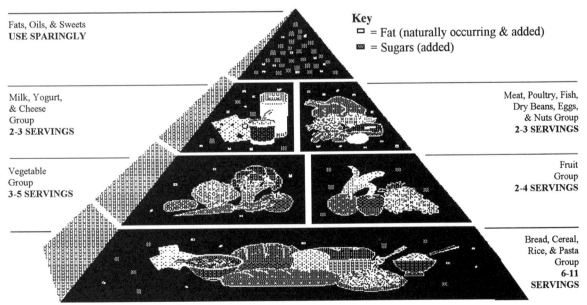

Source: U.S. Department of Agriculture & U.S. Department of Health and Human Services

Lesson Plans for Featured Book 3

Slawson, M. B. (1994). <u>Apple picking time</u>. New York: Crown Publishers.
A little girl goes with her family to pick apples at harvest time. After picking a long
time, she finally fills her whole bin and gets a mark on a ticket that she accomplished her
goal. Advanced reading level.

Pre-Reading Activities for *Apple Picking Time*

Brainstorm a list of community activities that bring people together. For example, parades, seasonal
festivals, emergencies (e.g., floods, tornados, hurricanes, earthquakes), and community clean-up days.
(MI = V/L)

Investigate the various food festivals in your county or region. Compare the festivals in other parts of
the state and country. Use e-mail to pen pal with another person to determine what festivals
occur and what makes them unique. For example, Ohio has a Black Walnut Festival, Sauerkraut
Festival, Pork Festival, Strawberry Festival, and Taste-of-City Festivals. Other states have Seafood
Festival (Lousiana, Alabama, and Florida), World Largest Apple Pie Festival (Kentucky), and others.
(MI = V/L, I/S)

Post-Reading Activities for *Apple Picking Time*

<u>Questions to develop thinking skills</u> (Bloom's Taxonomy)

1. Knowledge:	Name the people that encouraged the little girl throughout her day at the apple orchard.
2. Comprehension:	State the main idea of the story. Is the story about food?
3. Application:	Make a list of the many ways that apples can be used in the everyday life of a community.
4. Analysis:	Compare the number of half moons that Anna punched on her card at lunchtime with the number of half moons that her parents punched on their cards. What do the half moons represent?
5. Synthesis:	Imagine the feelings of the community members two days before the apple harvest begins, during the harvest, and two days after the harvest.
6. Evaluation:	Decide if the people in the community enjoyed the apple picking event. How would you recommend someone new to the community to participate?

Solo Work for *Apple Picking Time*

Bring an apple to school and share an adventure story about how the apple traveled to your classroom. Use your imagination on how you found and selected the apple. What color is it? What shape is it? Who bought or found the apple? What does it feel like in your hand? How do you think it will taste? How would you prepare it? Have students brainstorm additional questions of interest before sharing their apple adventures. (MI = V/L, B/K)

Small Group Work for *Apple Picking Time*

Complete the following phrases related to apples:
1) An apple a day....
2) An apple of your...
3) An apple for the...

Take these phrases home to your parents or caregivers to see how they complete the phrases. Record the different responses and share with your small group. Try to create additional slogans about apples. Make a bumper sticker of your favorite slogan for your bike or room. (MI = V/L, I/S, B/K)

Whole Class Work for *Apple Picking Time*

Organize a Community Share and Care Festival with other teachers and students in your building and/or district. Determine a location, date, and community advertisements for requesting donations of clothing and canned goods. Some students can prepare the posters and decorations. Other students can set prices for the donated products. Students can also make crafts and food for sale. Since Apple Picking Time is the theme book in this lesson, students might like to make apple projects and products for display or sale.

How can you educate your community about the apple as a nutritional food during your festival?
Have you eaten your five fruits and vegetables today for good nutrition and disease prevention?
See if the American Cancer Society or other health organization in your community will promote the National Cancer Institute's Five-a-Day Challenge during your festival. Learn more about it by visiting their website at http://cancernet.nci.nih.gov/occdocs/fiveday/tester.html

Why not ask health education classes at your local middle school and high school to assist with health-related booths and demonstrations? Maybe you can set up a computer booth so folks can use the 5 A Day Adventures CD-ROM program developed by Dole Food Company, Inc. in collaboration with the Society for Nutrition Education. Also check out the Pyramid Challenge CD-ROM for healthy eating. Both of these resources are found in the Teaching Resources at the end of this book. (MI = I/S, B/K, V/S, V/L)

If you want to add a really fun twist to your Community Share and Care Festival why not involve folks in a riddle contest about different foods? Good fun, food humor, and good food all add up to good health. Check out some sample riddles about different foods (Matthews & Robinson, 1993) in the Teaching Resources at the end of this book. (MI = V/L)

Across the Curriculum for *Apple Picking Time*
Social Studies
What do you know about migrant farmers? Does your community use migrant farmers for planting or harvesting crops. Investigate the role and needs of the migrant farmer in America. (MI = V/L)
Mathematics
Draw and cut apples out of red, green and yellow construction paper, or use real apples. Use three apples each. Cut the red apples in half, the yellow apples in quarters, and the green apples in thirds. Place all apple pieces in a basket. Count the pieces as a class and compare the number of servings available for each type of apple. (MI = B/K, L/M)
Science
Did you know that roses and apples are first cousins in the plant family? Any climate or country that can grow roses can also grow apples. Apples are our second most favorite fruit, with bananas taking center stage as the most favorite fruit. There are spring apples, fall apples, baking apples, eating apples, and some apples that seem only right for making applesauce. All apples contain fructose which gives them the special sweet flavor; fiber which gives us bulk in our diets; and pectin whose main purpose is to give apples a tart flavor. Eat a green or unripe apple. Does it feel like your apple gave "pucker power" to your cheeks? That is pectin. As the apple ripens the pectin is converted into fructose and it gains in sweetness and loses the pucker sensation. Pectin is a very useful compound (found in all unripe fruit) that can solidify carbohydrates. Pectin is used commercially and at home in jellies to make the jelly become firm and not runny. (MI = V/L)
Language Arts
Study the life and time of Johnny Appleseed. If you live in the Midwest, investigate if any of the older apple trees in your area were planted at the time of Johnny Appleseed. Locate at least five different picture books describing Johnny Appleseed's life. In small groups, compare and contrast the life of Johnny Appleseed in one of the books using a story map. List the title, author, setting, and characters of each story. Then list the beginning, middle, and end of each story. Share your findings with the whole class. (MI = I/S, V/L, V/S)
Physical Education
Reaching for apples on a tree requires a lot of stretching. It is important to stretch your muscles before physical activity. Pretend to reach for an apple on a tree. Hold the stretch without bouncing for 15 to 30 seconds, then relax. Repeat again. Stretching helps to develop your flexibility, and sometimes balance and coordination if you are on a ladder! (MI = B/K)
Art
Cut apples into thin slices to make either apple necklaces, wreaths or dolls. Dry and decorate. These creations can be used for display or sale at the Care-and-Share Festival. (MI = B/K, V/S)
Music
In the story, people are listening to the radio while picking apples. What music do you listen to when you are with your family? Do you change the type of music for different activities? What music do you play when you eat? Play some examples. (MI = V/L, M/R)

Across the Curriculum

Other Books to Read for
"Down on the Farm"

This list contains excellent books to read for learning about Down on the Farm. Use these books along with the Featured Books when teaching the lessons on the previous pages.

Altman, L. J. (1993). Amelia's road. New York: Lee & Low Books Inc.
    Amelia, the daughter of migrant farm workers, is tired of moving around and dreams of a permanent home. She finds a special place for herself so she doesn't feel so bad about leaving. The family continues to harvest peaches, apples, carrots, and tomatoes.

Creedle, E. (1934). Down down the mountain. New York: Elscuier/Nelson Books.
    Hetty and Hank want shoes, but Pappy says they have no money. So Granny gives them an idea how to raise the money. They grow some turnips to take down the mountain at harvest time. On the way to town, they give most of their turnips away to people who need them. With the one remaining turnip, Hetty and Hank win the top prize at the fair. They return home with a big story and new shoes.

Foster, D. V. (1961). A pocketful of seasons. New York: Lothrop, Lee and Shephard Books.
    A farmer tells Andy what happens to his crops from spring to winter.

Good, E. W. (1994). Fall is here! I love it! Intercourse, PA: Good Books.
    Fall is here! Leaves are falling off the trees, corn is being harvested, and the garden is being readied for the winter. Brilliant colors illustrate this wonderful story.

Good, E. W. (1990). It's summertime. Intercourse, PA: Good Books.
    It is summertime and the leaves are green. The berries are almost ripe-just a few more days. It's fun to walk barefoot in the grass and go swimming when it is warm outside!

Hall, Z. (1994). It's pumpkin time! New York: Scholastic Inc.
    Halloween is on its way, and it is time to plant the pumpkin seeds. A little girl and her brother plant the seeds and watch them grow. The shoots pop up, grow into vines, flowers bloom, and at last the pumpkins are ready to be picked!

Ipcar, D. (1976). Hard scrabble harvest. New York: Doubleday & Co., Inc.
    After the farmer plants his crops, he needs to keep a close eye on them. He puts up a scarecrow to scare the birds, then chases the chickens out of his field. When autumn comes, he harvests his crops and makes a big Thanksgiving dinner.

Krauss, R. (1989). The carrot seed. New York: Scholastic Inc.
    A little boy plants a carrot seed and takes good care of it. Even though his family tells him it won't grow, one day it finally does.

Other Books to Read,
Continued

Noble, T. H. (1984). <u>Apple tree christmas</u>. New York: Dial Books For Young Readers
It's time to make apple butter. When all the apples are picked, Katrina uses the tree as a playhouse. However, a blizzard occurs and Katrina's father must cut down the tree for firewood.

Nordgvist, S. (1985). <u>Pancake pie</u>. New York: Morrow Junior Books.
Festus, the farmer, wants to bake a cake for his cat's birthday. He has many obstacles to overcome to get the supplies to make the cake. Finally, he is able to make and eat the cake.

Pochocki, E. (1993). <u>The mushroom man</u>. New York: Simon & Schuster Books for Young Readers.
An old man, known as the mushroom man, works on a mushroom farm. People say that his head looks like a mushroom. They tease him and call him names. He befriends an even uglier animal, and they are happy together.

Rockwell, A. (1994). <u>Apples and pumpkins</u>. New York: Scholastic Inc.
A little girl goes with her parents to a farm where they pick apples and choose the best pumpkin for carving. At home, the family prepares for Halloween by carving the jack-o-lantern, dressing up, and going trick-or-treating.

Scheffler, U. (1990). <u>The giant apple</u>. Minneapolis: Carolrhoda Books, Inc.
Every year there is a festival where all the farmers bring their biggest vegetables. The same people win the prize for the biggest vegetables every year. The people of Appleville decide they will do everything possible to win. The next year they win the contest and have to eat apples all winter long because that is all they planted.

Titherington, J. (1990). <u>Pumpkin pumpkin</u>. New York: Scholastic Inc.
A little boy plants a pumpkin seed and watches it grow from a tiny sprout to a huge orange pumpkin. In the end, he picks the pumpkin and carves it for Halloween. However, he does save six seeds for planting next spring.

Wilder, L. I. (1994). <u>Winter days in the big woods</u>. New York: HarperCollins Children's Books.
Laura and her family prepare for winter as they harvest the potatoes, carrots, peas, onions, beets, turnips, cabbages, peppers and pumpkins. They store the food inside and they have plenty to eat all winter.

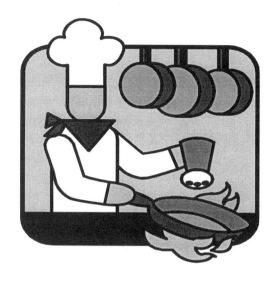

Letter to Food Service Professionals

We are starting a new adventure in learning called Cycle of Life. During this unit, we will be tasting different types of fruits and vegetables and different kinds of milk and cheeses. We may also make tortillas or nachos.

We would like to use the following equipment and supplies during the various festivals and food tastings we plan to have during this unit:

Refrigerator
Microwave Oven
Cutting boards
Space for Preparing the Foods
Cups or glasses
Large jars (for growing bean sprouts)

We also hope you will teach us about food commodities that are given to school food service from the United States Department of Agriculture (USDA). Thank you for helping us to coordinate learning experiences between our cafeteria, classroom, and community.

Thank you for helping us to learn!

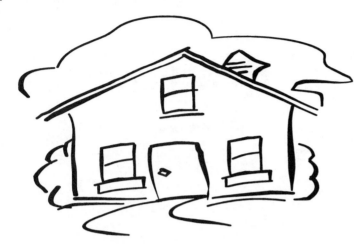

Letter to Parents and Caregivers

We are beginning a new nutrition and health unit called "Cycle of Life", which will include some cooking in the classroom and a food tasting. We will learn about different foods from Down on the Farm. Would you be willing to donate **one** of the items below for use during our unit? Anything you can do to help us by _____(date) will be greatly appreciated. We will also love your involvement during our classroom, cafeteria, and community activities.

- 1 gallon of whole milk
- 1 gallon 2% milk
- 1 quart buttermilk
- 1 gallon whole chocolate milk
- 1 gallon 2% chocolate milk
- 1 container (4 ounces) of cream cheese
- 1 container (4 ounces) of low fat cream cheese
- 1 container (4 ounces) of non-fat cream cheese
- 1 box of soda (plain) crackers
- 8 ounces of colby cheese
- 8 ounces of mozzarella cheese
- 8 ounces of munster cheese
- 1 stalk celery
- 1 bag of short carrots
- 2 ounces of oriental peas
- 1 small bunch of radishes
- 1 zuchinni
- 1 box of tooth picks
- 2 sacks of red apples
- 2 sacks of green apples
- 1 package of baked tortilla chips
- 1 package of tortilla shells

Thank you kindly!

For the Pleasure of Reading

This booklist can be sent home during Unit 4: Cycle of Life, so that your students and their families can read additional literature about food and nutrition together. You can also place these books in your classroom library during the unit. These books are considered secondary resources for this unit. Each book and its abstract is listed as a primary resource in another unit. Use the index at the back of this book to see how titles are crosslisted with other units. Our goal is to show how each book can be used in multiple ways to teach nutrition and health concepts.

Down on the Farm

Adoff, A. (1971). Ma nda la. New York: HarperCollins Children's Books.

Aylesworth, J. (1992). The folks in the valley. New York: HarperCollins Children's Books.

Bond, R. (1988). Cherry tree. Honesdale, PA: Boyds Hill Press.

Carle, E. (1992). Pancakes, pancakes! New York: Scholastic Inc.

dePaola, T. (1978). Pancakes for breakfast. San Diego: Scholastic Inc.

Ehlert, L. (1990). Growing vegetable soup. San Diego: Scholastic Inc.

Ericsson, J. (1993). No milk! New York: William Morrow & Co., Inc.

Gage, W. (1976). Squash pie. New York: Greenwillow Books.

Joosse, B. M. (1987). Jam day. New York: HarperCollins Children's Books.

Kelley, T. (1989). Let's eat. New York: Dutton Children's Books.

Kimmelman, L. (1989). Frannie's fruits. New York: HarperCollins Children's Books.

King, C. (1994). The vegetables go to bed. New York: Crown Publishers.

Lember, B. H. (1994). A book of fruit. New York: Ticknor and Fields Books.

Lottridge, C. (1990). One watermelon seed. New York: Oxford University Press, Inc.

MacDonald, E. (1990). Mr. macgregor's breakfast egg. New York: Penguin Group.

McNulty, F. (1987). The lady and the spider. New York: HarperCollins Children's Books.

Micucci, C. (1992). The life and the times of the apple. New York: Orchard Books.

Mitchell, B., & Sandford, J. (1993). Down buttermilk lane. New York: Lothrop, Lee and Shepard

Obligado, L. (1993). The chocolate cow. New York: Simon & Schuster Books for Young Readers.

Palmisciano, D. (1989). Garden partners. New York: Antheneum Books for Young Readers.

Polacco, P. (1993). The bee tree. New York: Philomel Books.

Priceman, M. (1994). How to make an apple pie and see the world. New York: Knopf Books.

Rice, E. (1990). At grammy's house. New York: Greenwillow Books.

Steffy, J. (1987). The school picnic. Intercourse, PA: Good Books.

Williams, S. A. (1992). Working cotton. New York: Harcourt Brace & Co.

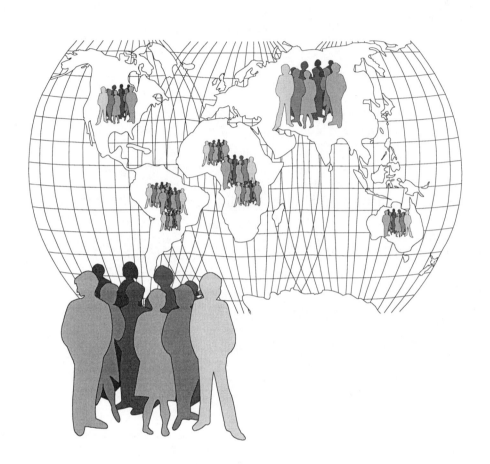

Unit 5:
<u>World of People</u>

Multigenerational Gatherings
Multicultural Connections

Unit 5: World of People

Instructional activities for Unit 5 have been designed to achieve the *National Health Education Standards* as shown in bold-face type:

⟹ 1. **Students will comprehend concepts related to health promotion and disease prevention.**
   Performance Indicators. As a result of health instruction in Grades K-4, students will
   6. Identify health problems that should be detected and treated early.
   7. Explain how childhood injuries and illnesses can be prevented or treated.

⟹ 4. **Students will analyze the influence of culture, media, technology, and other factors on health.**
   Performance Indicators. As a result of health instruction in Grades K-4, students will
   1. Describe how culture influences personal health behaviors.
   4. Explain how information from school and family influences health.

⟹ 5. **Students will demonstrate the ability to use interpersonal communication skills to enhance health.**
   Performance Indicators. As a result of health instruction in Grades K-4, students will
   2. describe characteristics needed to be a responsible friend and family member.
   3. demonstrate healthy ways to express needs, wants, and feelings.
   4. demonstrate ways to communicate care, consideration, and respect of self & others.
   5. demonstrate attentive listening skills to build and maintain healthy relationships.

⟹ 6. **Students will demonstrate the ability to use goal setting and decision-making skills to enhance health.**
   Performance Indicators. As a result of health instruction in Grades K-4, students will
   1. demonstrate the ability to apply a decision-making process to health issues and problems.
   3. predict outcomes of positive health decisions.

⟹ 7. **Students will demonstrate the ability to advocate for personal, family, and community health.**
   Performance Indicators. As a result of health instruction in Grades K-4, students will
   3. identify community agencies that advocate for healthy individuals, families, & communitities.

| Unit 5: World of People |
| Scope & Sequence of Nutrition Content |

Nutrition Content: Dietary Guidelines	Dumpling Soup	Valerie and the Silver Pear	Chicken Sunday	Halmoni and the Picnic	Knoxville, Tennessee	Too Many Tamales	The Relatives Came
Eat a variety of foods	X				X		X
Balance food with exercise		X		X	X		
Choose grains, vegetables, and fruits	X	X	X	X	X	X	X
Choose low fat and low cholesterol			X				X
Choose moderate sugars		X					X
Choose moderate salt/sodium				X			

Nutrition Content: Food Groups	Dumpling Soup	Valerie and the Silver Pear	Chicken Sunday	Halmoni and the PIcnic	Knoxville, Tennessee	Too Many Tamales	The Relatives Came
Bread, Cereal, Rice, & Pasta Group	X		X	X	X	X	X
Fruit Group	X	X					X
Vegetable Group	X		X	X	X		
Milk, Yogurt, & Cheese Group					X		
Meat, Poultry, Fish, Beans, Eggs, & Nuts Group	X		X	X	X	X	
Fats, Oils, & Sweets Group		X	X				

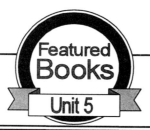

Featured Books
Unit 5

Overall Featured Book for Unit 5

Rattigan, J. K. (1993). <u>Dumpling</u> <u>soup</u>. New York: Little, Brown & Co.

> Marisa, a little girl who lives in Hawaii, helps to make dumplings this year. Her relatives travel from all over Hawaii to come for a New Year's celebration. They all bring food and are excited to eat the dumpling soup that Marisa helped prepare. Advanced reading level.

Books for Focused Theme: Multigenerational Gatherings

Darling, B. (1992). <u>Valerie</u> <u>and</u> <u>the</u> <u>silver</u> <u>pear</u>. New York: Macmillan Children's Book Group.

> Valerie enjoys visiting her grandfather. One day, during her visit, he tells her a story of a pear tree. After hearing the story, they decide to make pear pies. Intermediate reading level.

Polacco, P. (1992). <u>Chicken</u> <u>sunday</u>. New York: Scholastic Inc.

> The children want to buy an Easter bonnet for their cook, Miss Eula, but they don't have any money. They discover a way to earn the money for Miss Eula. She cries when they give her the bonnet. Advanced reading Level.

Choi, S. N. (1993). <u>Halmoni</u> <u>and</u> <u>the</u> <u>picnic</u>. Boston: Houghton Mifflin Co.

> Yunmi's grandmother moves from Korea to New York City and is not used to American traditions. Yunmi worries that other people will make fun of her grandmother. Advanced reading level.

Books for Focused Theme: Multicultural Connections

Giovanni, N. (1994). <u>Knoxville</u>, <u>tennessee</u>. New York: Scholastic, Inc.

> A young girl likes summer best because of the fresh corn from her daddy's garden; the okra, barbecue; and homemade ice cream from the church picnic; and the gospel music from the church homecoming. She also likes to go the mountains with her grandmother where she feels safe and warm. Beginning reading level.

Soto, G., & Martinez, E. (1993). <u>Too</u> <u>many</u> <u>tamales</u>. New York: Putnam Publishing Group.

> Maria is excited because it is Christmas Eve and she is helping her family make tamales for the holiday. When Maria's mom leaves the kitchen, Maria tries on her mom's ring. Maria thinks she loses the ring in the tamale mix and tries to find it. Intermediate reading level.

Rylant, C. (1985). <u>The relatives came.</u> New York: Macmillan Children's Book Group.

> Relatives visit from Virginia and bring lots of laughter, hugs, food, and good times. During the reunion, they eat, sleep, and breathe together. Intermediate reading level.

<table>
<tr><td>

Overall Featured Book
of
Unit 5: World of People

</td><td>

Dumpling Soup
by Jama Kim Rattigan
Little, Brown & Company, 1993

</td></tr>
</table>

This lesson addresses the following Dietary Guidelines for Americans:

⇒   *1. Eat a variety of foods.*

      2. Balance the food you eat with physical activity; maintain or improve your weight.

⇒   *3. Choose a diet with plenty of grain products, vegetables, and fruits.*

      4. Choose a diet low in fat, saturated fat, and cholesterol.

      5. Choose a diet moderate in sugars.

      6. Choose a diet moderate in salt and sodium.

      7. Choose an alcohol and drug-free lifestyle.

This lesson highlights the following food groups from the Food Guide Pyramid:

⇒   *Bread, Cereal, Rice, & Pasta Group*

⇒   *Fruit Group*

⇒   *Vegetable Group*

      Milk, Yogurt, & Cheese Group

⇒   *Meat, Poultry, Fish, Dry Beans, Eggs, & Nuts Group*

Food Guide Pyramid
A Guide to Daily Food Choices

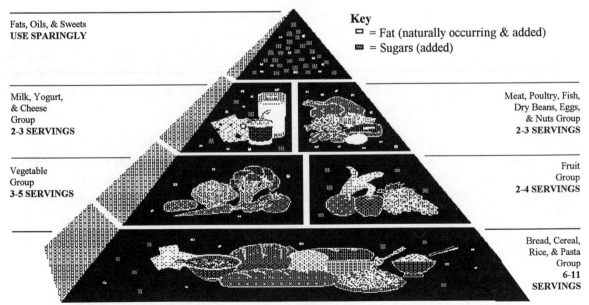

Source: U.S. Department of Agriculture & U.S. Department of Health and Human Services

Lesson Plans for Overall Feature Book

Rattigan, J. K. (1993). <u>Dumpling</u> <u>soup</u>. New York: Little, Brown & Co.
Marisa, a little girl who lives in Hawaii, helps to make dumplings this year. Her relatives travel from all over Hawaii to come for a New Year's celebration. They all bring food and are excited to eat the dumpling soup that Marisa helped prepare. Advanced reading level.

Pre-Reading Activities for *Dumpling Soup*

Find on a world map the countries of Japan, Korea, China, and Hawaiian Islands. Discuss the concept of Oriental New Year using the publisher's note at the front of the book. (MI = V/S, V/L)

Describe some special celebration or tradition that your family has during the New Year holiday. (MI = V/S)

Post-Reading Activities

<u>Questions to develop thinking skills</u> (Bloom's Taxonomy)

1. Knowledge: Tell and show the different ways that dumplings were wrapped in the book.

2. Comprehension: Review and explain the various dishes that Marisa and her family ate at their New Year's Eve celebration.

3. Application: Put in order the events of the New Year's Eve celebration. Is it wise for Marisa and the other children to participate in those events every night? Why or why not?

4. Analysis: Categorize the foods eaten by Marisa's family on New Year's Eve into the Five Food Groups. Did they eat a well balanced meal?

5. Synthesis: Imagine how many hours over how many days it took Marisa's family to create their dumpling soup. Change the story so it can happen in one day.

6. Evaluation: Recommend a change in your New Year's Eve celebration after reading the book. Decide if the change will be easy or hard to do with your family.

Solo Work for *Dumpling Soup* (MI = B/K)

Teacher:

- Buy, chop and mix bok choy, cabbage, onions, celery, garlic and cooked chicken (diced, home prepared, or out of a can). Put mixture into a covered container and transport to school.
- Buy two egg roll wrappers (dough usually found in vegetable section) per person.
- Buy wax paper and tear 12 inch pieces for each student.
- Set up work stations for making dumplings. Place container of dumpling mixture and a small bowl of water on a large tray. Place egg roll wrappers on a second tray to be used as a work space.
- Locate a hot plate and a pot for boiling the dumplings.
- Demonstrate how to make a dumpling to the entire class, then invite one student at a time to the work station to make two dumplings each.

Students:

- Wash hands with soap and warm running water after your teacher demonstrates how to do it.
- Place a fresh piece of wax paper on the tray at your work space.
- Place an egg roll wrapper on the wax paper.
- Place a tablespoon of dumpling mixture onto a wrapper.
- Wrap the dough over the mixture.
- Dab a little water over the seam and pinch the seam with your fingers.
- Place your dumpling in a large storage container.
- Make one more dumpling.

Teacher:

- Place all of the dumplings into boiling water. The dumplings are cooked when they bounce to the surface. The dumplings will look dull and wrinkled.
- Cover the dumplings with foil and set aside until banquet time.

Small Group Work for *Dumpling Soup* (MI = B/K, V/S)

Teacher:

- Buy fresh oranges, bananas, apples, or other fruit in season. Also buy canned pineapple or fresh pineapple if precut.
- Buy colorful toothpicks.

Students:

- Wash, peel, and cut the fruit.
- Arrange the fruit on plates and insert toothpicks for a celebration dinner.

Teacher:

- Obtain and cook instant rice, or steam rice in a rice cooker.

Students:

- Let the students mix honey and rice (optional nuts and dates) to form small round cakes called moon cakes or Yak pap.
- Arrange the moon cakes on plates.

Whole Class Work for *Dumpling Soup* (MI = B/K, V/L, I/I, I/S)

Sit, eat, and enjoy. During the meal, discuss the different ways that you might celebrate holidays in your house. Who visits? Who helps to prepare the food? What types of food do you eat? What type of music is played? What kind of games or fun activities do you do? How long do your guests stay?

Across the Curriculum for *Dumpling Soup*

Social Studies

Practice vocabulary words from the glossary of *Dumpling Soup*. Make flashcards for the Korean words and label items in the classroom during the unit. Invite family members to class who can discuss personal stories about an Oriental New Year. Nutrition is more than just food to eat. Nutrition also deals with the styles of eating. The main characters in the book used chop sticks to handle their food. Larger chop sticks would be used to place food from the large serving dishes to individual plates. A family in Morocco would use spoons and their fingers to consume their meals. They would all share one large platter with no individual plates. There is a feeling in the Morocoan society that this helps to maintain a very strong family tradition. In most American families, there are serving bowls and individual plates for each person. This is known as Family Style of food service. The Russians and Swedish are credited with the "moving board" or smorgasbord. It is known now as buffet style. When first invented a servant would carry a long board with many different foods on it. People would stand and eat from the board as the servant carried it. Now the board is stationary and the people move around it. What type of food service does your school have? What kind of food service style do you practice at home? (MI = V/L)

Mathematics

Count different kinds of shoes that students are wearing in your class and graph them. Classify shoes by color, style, and use. Incorporate basic arthrimetic skills in the process. (MI = L/M, V/S)

Language Arts

Think about a time when you were the first person awake in your house. Tell a partner what you saw, heard, felt, sensed, and smelled. The partner should write the ideas on a piece of paper. Reverse roles while one person talks and the other person writes. Next, describe why you were up before the others in your family. Discuss how your sleep patterns may change when you have out-of- town guests staying with you. (MI = V/L, I/I, I/S)

Physical Education

Walk around the room as if you are wearing thongs. How would you walk in a pair of shoes that are way too big? How would you walk in a pair of heavy boots? What about ice skates? Roller blades? Running shoes? How would you walk if the room was full of jello? Peanut butter? Walk in a different direction. (Skills developed: creative movement with different effort, force, direction, and pathways). (MI = B/K)

Art

Design your own sandals out of paper and cardboard by using the examples shown in the book. Display them in your classroom. Make tropical trees out of cardboard tubes and green construction paper to decorate your room during the unit. (MI = V/S)

Music

Play Oriental music during the banquet. Investigate the different instruments that are used in Oriental music. Display pictures of the instruments or some of the actual instruments in your classroom. (MI = M/R, V/S)

Across the Curriculum

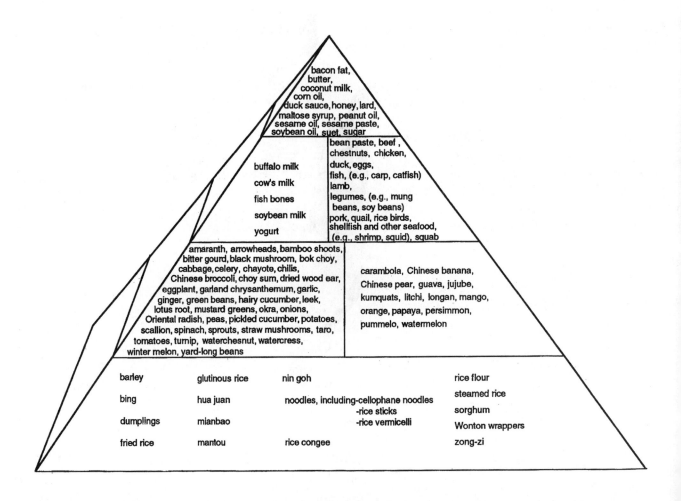

bacon fat,
butter,
coconut milk,
corn oil,
duck sauce, honey, lard,
maltose syrup, peanut oil,
sesame oil, sesame paste,
soybean oil, suet, sugar

buffalo milk

cow's milk

fish bones

soybean milk

yogurt

bean paste, beef ,
chestnuts, chicken,
duck, eggs,
fish, (e.g., carp, catfish)
lamb,
legumes, (e.g., mung
beans, soy beans)
pork, quail, rice birds,
shellfish and other seafood,
(e.g., shrimp, squid), squab

amaranth, arrowheads, bamboo shoots,
bitter gourd, black mushroom, bok choy,
cabbage, celery, chayote, chilis,
Chinese broccoli, choy sum, dried wood ear,
eggplant, garland chrysanthemum, garlic,
ginger, green beans, hairy cucumber, leek,
lotus root, mustard greens, okra, onions,
Oriental radish, peas, pickled cucumber, potatoes,
scallion, spinach, sprouts, straw mushrooms, taro,
tomatoes, turnip, waterchesnut, watercress,
winter melon, yard-long beans

carambola, Chinese banana,
Chinese pear, guava, jujube,
kumquats, litchi, longan, mango,
orange, papaya, persimmon,
pummelo, watermelon

barley	glutinous rice	nin goh		rice flour
bing	hua juan	noodles, including-cellophane noodles		steamed rice
		-rice sticks		sorghum
dumplings	mianbao	-rice vermicelli		Wonton wrappers
fried rice	mantou	rice congee		zong-zi

Chinese American Foods
and the Food Guide Pyramid

Source: 1993 *Pyramid Packet*, Penn State Nutrition Center,
5 Henderson Building, University Park, PA 16802; (814) 865-6323.

Focused Theme:
Multigenerational Gatherings

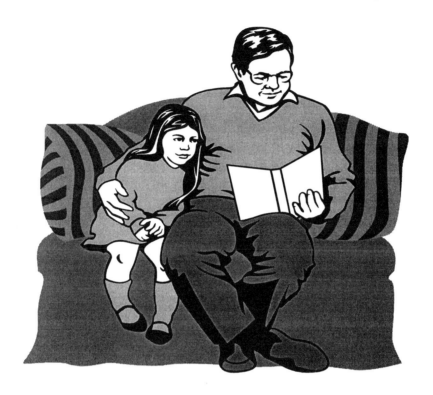

Overview of Multigenerational Gatherings

This focused theme highlights the social gatherings we share with people from our families and friends who are from an older generation. We gain a healthy perspective on aging when we share thoughts, feelings, past memories, and current events with people of all ages. Several featured books in this unit show what it's like to grow up with the love and support of people from many generations while sharing everyday activities like meal preparation and eating.

*Featured Book #1
of the Focused Theme:
Multigenerational
Gatherings*

Valerie and the Silver Pear
by Benjamin Darling
Four Winds Press, 1992

This lesson addresses the following Dietary Guidelines for Americans:

1. Eat a variety of foods.
⇒ 2. *Balance the food you eat with physical activity; maintain or improve your weight.*
⇒ 3. *Choose a diet with plenty of grain products, vegetables, and fruits.*
4. Choose a diet low in fat, saturated fat, and cholesterol.
⇒ 5. *Choose a diet moderate in sugars.*
6. Choose a diet moderate in salt and sodium.
7. Choose an alcohol and drug-free lifestyle.

This lesson highlights the following food groups from the Food Guide Pyramid:

Bread, Cereal, Rice, & Pasta Group
⇒ *Fruit Group*
Vegetable Group
Milk, Yogurt, & Cheese Group
Meat, Poultry, Fish, Dry Beans, Eggs, & Nuts Group
⇒ *Fats, Oils, & Sweets*

Food Guide Pyramid
A Guide to Daily Food Choices

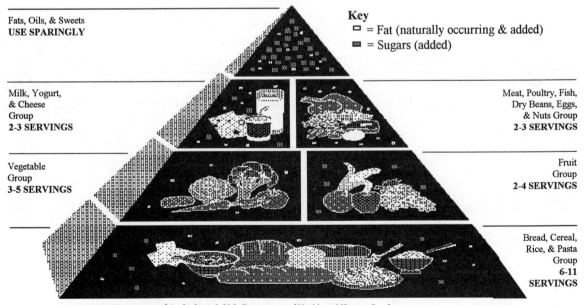

Source: U.S. Department of Agriculture & U.S. Department of Health and Human Services

Lesson Plans for Featured Book 1

Darling, B. (1992). <u>Valerie</u> <u>and</u> <u>the</u> <u>silver</u> <u>pear</u>. New York: Macmillan Children's Book.
Valerie enjoys visiting her grandfather. One day, during her visit, he tells her a story of a pear tree. After hearing the story, they decide to make pear pies. Intermediate reading level.

Pre-Reading Activities for *Valerie and the Silver Pear*

Take a field trip to an orchard to learn how fruit trees are cared for and how fruit is harvested. You might even visit a berry farm where raspberries, blueberries, or strawberries are grown to compare the difference. (MI = B/K, V/L)

Ask grandparents or an older person to tell a story about their favorite cooking, baking, or eating experience. Bring a recipe or momento to class to use when retelling their story. Have five students share their stories each day when you work on the focused theme of multigenerational gatherings. (MI = V/L, I/I)

Post-Reading Activities for *Valerie and the Silver Pear*

<u>Questions to develop thinking skills</u> (Bloom's Taxonomy)

1. Knowledge: Name the three different fruit trees found in grandpa's garden and which fruit he might have liked the best.

2. Comprehension: Explain why Valerie and her grandpa called the librarian while making the pear pie.

3. Application: Put in order the six steps needed for making a pear pie.

4. Analysis: In the story, Valerie followed a recipe to make the pies. Write a recipe for making your favorite sandwich. Test your recipe and see if it works. Compare the similarities and differences between two different recipes.

5. Synthesis: What if Valerie and her grandpa *had* found a silver pear? What would they have done? Who would they have given it to?

6. Evaluation: Revise the story and use apples instead of pears to make the pies. Summarize the events from picking the apples to eating the pie.

Solo Work for *Valerie and the Silver Pear*

Write about a special time *you* shared with a grandparent or an older person. How did you celebrate the time together? If your celebration included food, be sure to describe the food you ate. Use descriptive words to explain the food's color, shape, texture, taste, and smell. Mail or deliver a copy of your memories to your grandparent or older friend. If your grandparent or older friend is no longer living, share your special memories with someone who knew them. How can we keep memories alive about special people in our lives? (MI = I/I, V/L)

Small Group Work for *Valerie and the Silver Pear*

Investigate the different living arrangements at retirement centers in your community. What kinds of questions would you ask people who live in retirement homes? Compare living arrangements between different people at a retirement home. Can the residents still prepare their own meals? How do they like the arrangement? How do they go to the grocery store? Do they have to prepare all of their meals or can they eat at the dining hall when they feel like it? How does eating change when you get older? Are there special considerations needed when fixing food for older persons? What kind of food gifts have the residents received from their family members or friends? Share what you learned with your class.
(MI = V/L, I/S)

Whole Class Work for *Valerie and the Silver Pear*

Based on your work in small groups, decide if your class would be willing to plan a pie baking day at a local retirement center or retirement home. What arrangements will need to be made for transporting your class to the retirement center or home? With whom do you discuss the possibilities for setting up a work space for cutting the fruit for a pie, filling commercially prepared pie crusts, and baking the pies? What can you learn from the older persons about baking pies? Serving the pies? How can the food service professionals in the kitchen help your day go smoothly? What donations can you receive from local food markets and community service agencies to offset any costs for the day? Perhaps you can even ask your retired friends to help name the special event! (MI = V/L, I/S, B/K)

Across the Curriculum for *Valerie and the Silver Pear*

Social Studies
Research the history of different fruits that are grown on trees and grown on bushes. Draw a map with a legend to show where each of these fruits are grown. (MI = V/L, V/S)

Mathematics
Look through nursery and seed catalogs to find out how many different kinds of fruit trees you can grow. Make a table to compare costs, length of growing time, and how many years before it produces fruit. (MI = V/S, V/L, L/M)

Science
Did you ever eat a very good pear? Remember how it was soft, sweet, and seemed to just melt in your mouth? Now did you ever bite into a very bad pear? Remember how it felt in your mouth with the lumps and grains of material? The difference in quality was the texture of the fiber. Fruit contains a high percentage of fiber. Fiber cannot be digested by the human body. Termites are the only creatures on earth that can digest fiber. Termites can eat wood from your pencil or your house and mechanically and chemically turn the wood into glucose. Even though your body can not turn this fiber into glucose, you still need the fiber for bulk in your diet. Fiber helps the waste material move quickly through your small intestines and colon, which helps prevent constipation. Go on the World Wide Web to learn about the Take 5 A Day Challenge from the National Cancer Institute. Access it @ http://cancernet.nci.nih.gov/occdocs/fiveday/tester.html
Why should we eat fresh fruits and vegetables? (MI = V/L)

Language Arts
Look in your local phone book for names of fruit orchards or berry farms in your area. Create a list of names for a new fruit orchard or berry farm. Choose one of the names and write ten sentences that describe one of the jobs you might have at the orchard or berry farm. (MI = V/L)

Physical Education
Choreograph a creative dance about trees in an orchard. Some tree movements can show growth and branching out and other movements can show a tree in a storm. What can you do in trees to develop your physical fitness? Talk about climbing trees, swinging from a tire or swing, and reading a book under a shade tree. How do these activities compare? (MI = B/K, M/R)

Art
Draw an orchard in any season that you choose. How does your composition compare in line and form to another student's composition? (MI = V/S, V/L)

Music
Create a food jingle that can be used on a television commercial for a fruit or fruit product. You can even make an advertisement for the fruit orchard or berry farm you named in your Language Arts assignment above. (MI = M/R)

Across the Curriculum

*Featured Book #2
of the Focused Theme:
Multigenerational
Gatherings*

Chicken Sunday
by Patricia Polacco
Philomel Books, 1992

This lesson addresses the following Dietary Guidelines for Americans:
1. Eat a variety of foods.
2. Balance the food you eat with physical activity; maintain or improve your weight.
⇒ *3. Choose a diet with plenty of grain products, vegetables, and fruits.*
⇒ *4. Choose a diet low in fat, saturated fat, and cholesterol.*
5. Choose a diet moderate in sugars.
6. Choose a diet moderate in salt and sodium.
7. Choose an alcohol and drug-free lifestyle.

This lesson highlights the following food groups from the Food Guide Pyramid:
⇒ *Bread, Cereal, Rice, & Pasta Group*
Fruit Group
⇒ *Vegetable Group*
Milk, Yogurt, & Cheese Group
⇒ *Meat, Poultry, Fish, Dry Beans, Eggs, & Nuts Group*
⇒ *Fats, Oils, & Sweets*

Food Guide Pyramid
A Guide to Daily Food Choices

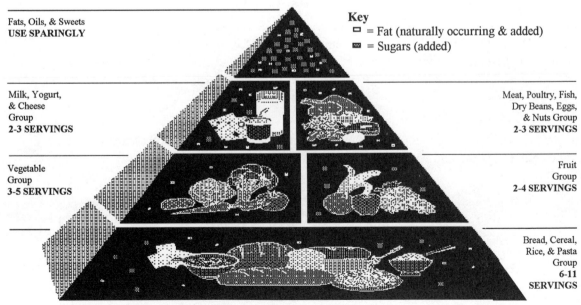

Source: U.S. Department of Agriculture & U.S. Department of Health and Human Services

Lesson Plans for Feature Book 2

Polacco, P. (1992). <u>Chicken</u> <u>sunday</u>. New York: Scholastic Inc.
The children want to buy an Easter bonnet for their cook, Miss Eula, but they don't have any money. They discover a way to earn the money for Miss Eula. She cries when they give her the bonnet. Advanced reading Level.

Pre-Reading Activities for *Chicken Sunday*

Brainstorm a list of friends and family members you know by name. Write each name on an index card. Ask students to sort the cards by gender first. Count the number of cards in each stack. Next sort the cards by different ages. Select three age groups to consider. Count the number of cards in each stack. Finally sort the cards by different culture ethnicities. Count the number of cards in different cultural groups. Discuss diversity in families and friendships. (MI = V/L, V/S, I/I)

Talk about the composition of different types (structures) of families in your classroom. Compare similarities and differences among students. (MI = V/L)

Post-Reading Activities for *Chicken Sunday*

Questions to develop thinking skills (Bloom's Taxonomy)

1. Knowledge: Tell why this book is titled *Chicken Sunday.*

2. Comprehension: Explain the different ways the characters used eggs in this story.

3. Application: Report another way that the children could prove themselves to Mr. Kodinski instead of by painting eggs.

4. Analysis: Examine the relationship between Patricia, Stewart, and Winston. Despite their physical and cultural differences, what helps them to maintain their friendship?

5. Synthesis: Change or improve the preparation of the Chicken Sunday dinner.

6. Evaluation: Decide if the author succeeded in showing the good values of the children?

Solo Work for *Chicken Sunday*

Make a fan for use at a class style show. Draw colorful foods from one food group on a 11 x 14 piece of paper. Fold the paper in one-inch lengths to form an accordian effect. Secure one end of the paper with tape and a rubber band. Spread the paper open to make a fan. Students can make fruit fans, vegetable fans, bread fans, meat fans, or milk fans. A minimum of five different foods should be drawn on the fans to represent one food group. Popsicle sticks can be used to make a sturdier handle for the fans. (MI = V/S)

Small Group Work for *Chicken Sunday*

Create a fancy hat to wear in a style show. Determine the colors, style, and decorations for a hat. Will it resemble a sun hat, baseball cap, or a hat that Miss Eula might wear? Choose one member of your group to model the hat. What determines good posture for modeling? Can posture be improved? Help your model practice good posture wearing your group's fancy hat. Take turns so everyone understands how to model. How does facial expression play a role in modeling? Write a descriptive script about your model's hat to be read at the style show. Don't forget to mention the designers' names. (MI = V/S, V/L, B/K, I/S)

Whole Class Work for *Chicken Sunday*

Color and decorate eggs (real or plaster of paris) to auction off during the style show. The auction will be based on the number of points that the students have earned during the week for good attendance, using good manners, completing assignments, eating breakfast each morning, and other positive behaviors. At the end of the week, students can tally their points, which determines how much they can "bid" for decorated eggs at the style show. Points can be placed on bid cards for each student. Ask an independent panel of people like secretaries, principals, and food service professionals from your school to assign points to the eggs. Make the points reasonable so that every student can "buy" at least one egg with their points. Students will turn in their point cards to buy the egg that they want.

Invite an auctioneer to the egg auction and style show to serve as the announcer, or ask an administrator from you school to serve in that role. Prepare a printed program for distribution at the event. Also design and send invitations to parents, grandparents, or guardians. Admission to the event will be one dozen cookies. Serve decaffeinated tea with the cookies. Hold the event in the cafeteria. Ask the food service professionals in your school to help with tablecloths, cookie trays, and other necessary supplies. Visitors can use the food fans during the style show to add a fun atmosphere to the day. (MI = B/K, V/S, L/M, V/L, I/S)

Across the Curriculum for *Chicken Sunday*

Social Studies

When the children had tea with the old man, they drank tea from tea cups and ate cookies. One of the pictures in the book shows a samovar for making tea in the girl's kitchen. The English have a formal tea with sandwiches, cake, or tea biscuits. Research other cultures that drink tea as a beverage. Compare their traditions. (MI = V/S, V/L)

Mathematics

Foods such as saurkraut, tamalas, spaghetti, apple pie, and okra were all brought to this country from other countries. This food culture enriches our own lives and helps us identify with our heritage. Ask a family member about your family heritage. America has been called a melting pot and more recently called a salad bowl. What foods have your ancestors added to the salad bowl of diversity? Make a large chart showing the number and variety of foods represented by different cultures in your class. (MI = V/L, I/S, L/M, V/S)

Science

Investigate what happens to eggs when they are hardboiled. Compare the results when you boil the eggs in a saucepan versus when you steam the eggs in a commercial egg cooker. To boil the eggs, place the eggs in a sauce pan and cover with water. Bring water to a boil, then put the lid on the pan and remove from the stove. Let eggs sit for 20 minutes, then drain the hot water off and exchange with cold water. Why should hardboiled eggs be submerged in cold water after cooking? Why can eggs boiled this way be hard to peel? A commercial egg cooker uses a puncture hole in the end of each egg before steaming. This hole helps to break the membrane of the egg shell. (MI = B/K, L/M)

Language Arts

Do a character study of different people in the story. Create a chart with the following headings: Who? Did what? When? Where? Why? New vocabulary? (MI = V/L, V/S)

Physical Education

Eggs were thrown in the story. Let's use a foam ball or yarn ball instead. Draw two target boards on the chalk board or make two out of cardboard. Divide students into two groups and give each group a ball. Each student should try to hit the highest point score on the target. Stand sideways to the target when preparing to throw the ball. Turn hips while in motion and step towards the target with the foot closest to the target, e.g., step with the left foot if right handed or vice versa. Individual scores can be tallied for a group score. (MI = V/S, B/K)

Art

Notice the real photographs that the author illustrator, Patricia Polacco, uses in the story. Share a photograph of yourself when you were younger with the class. Display the photograph in a picture frame or make a frame for your picture during art class. Arrange and display these photos in the cafeteria during the style show and auction. (MI = V/S)

Music

Choose a variety of songs to play during the style show. Select different styles of music to accompany the modeling of each hat. How does the tempo of the music effect the rate of movement by the model? (MI = M/R, B/K)

Across the Curriculum

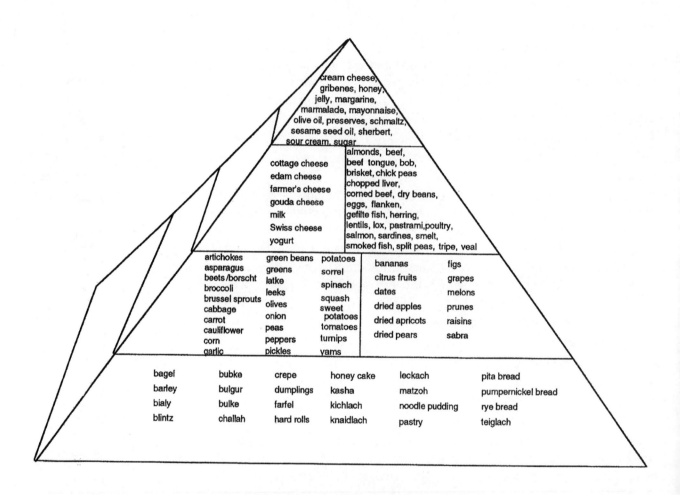

Jewish American Foods
and the Food Guide Pyramid

Source: 1993 *Pyramid Packet*, Penn State Nutrition Center,
5 Henderson Building, University Park, PA 16802; (814) 865-6323.

*Featured Book #3
of the Focused Theme:
Multigenerational
Gatherings*

Halmoni and the Picnic
by Sook Nyal Choi
Houghton Mifflin Co., 1993

This lesson addresses the following Dietary Guidelines for Americans:

1. Eat a variety of foods.
⇒ *2. Balance the food you eat with physical activity; maintain or improve your weight.*
⇒ *3. Choose a diet with plenty of grain products, vegetables, and fruits.*
4. Choose a diet low in fat, saturated fat, and cholesterol.
5. Choose a diet moderate in sugars.
⇒ *6. Choose a diet moderate in salt and sodium.*
7. Choose an alcohol and drug-free lifestyle.

This lesson highlights the following food groups from the Food Guide Pyramid:

⇒ *Bread, Cereal, Rice, & Pasta Group*
   Fruit Group
⇒ *Vegetable Group*
   Milk, Yogurt, & Cheese Group
⇒ *Meat, Poultry, Fish, Dry Beans, Eggs, & Nuts Group*

Food Guide Pyramid
A Guide to Daily Food Choices

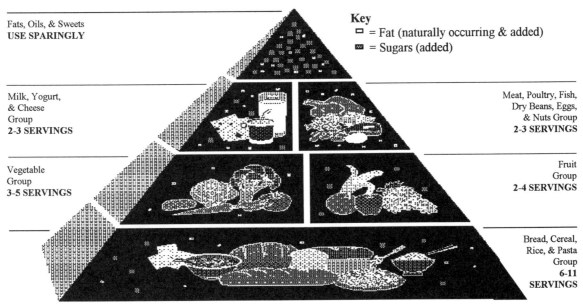

Source: U.S. Department of Agriculture & U.S. Department of Health and Human Services

Lesson Plans for Focused Theme 2

Choi, S. N. (1993). <u>Halmoni</u> <u>and</u> <u>the</u> <u>picnic</u>. Boston: Houghton Mifflin Co.
Yunmi's grandmother moves from Korea to New York City and is not used to American traditions. Yunmi worries that other people will make fun of her grandmother. Advanced reading level.

Pre-Reading Activities for *Halmoni and the Picnic*

Remember a time in your life when you had to move from your home, community, or country. Or think about a time when you changed schools, churches, or scouting troups. How did you cope with the change in your life? Explain your feelings then and your feelings now. (MI = I/I, V/L)

Name some coping skills that you used that were helpful at the time. Does everyone use the same coping skills in times of change? What are some helpful tips that you can share with others who are going through changes in their lives? (MI = I/I, V/L, I/S)

Post-Reading Activities for *Halmoni and the Picnic*

<u>Questions to develop thinking skills</u> (Bloom's Taxonomy)

1. *Knowledge:*   Remember what Halmoni made for the picnic. Turn and tell one person in class what she brought. Tell what Halmoni does instead of saying hello to Yunmi's friends.

2. *Comprehension:*   Explain why Halmoni is sad and shy at the beginning of the book. How do Yunmi and her friends try to help?

3. *Application:*   Do you know someone who is from another country? Role play how they are different in what they eat, wear, and act.

4. *Analysis:*   Compare life in the United States to life in Korea. Observe how Halmoni is different in clothing, food choices, mannerisms, and other things.

5. *Synthesis:*   Imagine if you were visiting another country where they ate different foods. Would you try foods from that country? What foods from the United States would you introduce to your foreign friends?

6. *Evaluation:*   Decide what will happen if Yunmi's grandmother chaperones next year's picnic. Do you think she will have the same customs and mannerisms? Recommend a different conclusion to the story.

Solo Work for *Halmoni and the Picnic*

Interview the oldest living member of your family in person, by mail, or over the telephone. Make a list of traditions or customs that your grandparents or great-grandparents used to do that you no longer practice today. Present these ideas verbally to your class. Then write a paragraph to describe how you are related to this person. (MI = I/S, V/L)

Small Group Work for *Halmoni and the Picnic*

Group students according to ethnicity or cultural backgrounds in class. Each group will research the food customs of their heritage by collecting recipes. Students are encouraged to obtain these recipes from family members, but library research in cookbooks can be done too. Each small group will write out recipe cards then tally whether the ingredients would be found in the bread group, vegetable group, fruit group, milk group, or meat group. Each small group agrees upon the one recipe to be shared with the food service professionals in the school. Each group should vote for the most balanced recipe, meaning the food that utilizes more than one food group in its ingredients.   (MI = I/S, V/L, B/K, L/M)

Whole Class Work for *Halmoni and the Picnic*

In cooperation with a food service professional in your school and/or registered dietitian, try to have a dietary analysis done of each of the selected recipes from the small group work. Compare the nutrient values of the different foods. What generalizations can be made about foods from the different cultures? Choose one of the foods and have a banquet in class like Halmoni did with the third grade students. Is there a family member from your classroom who would like to share the selected food or help prepare the selected food with your students? Let the class decide if this feast should be planned for your classroom, your cafeteria, a picnic or park, a local restaurant, or field trip to someone's home. (MI = L/M, V/L, B/K)

Across the Curriculum for *Halmoni and the Picnic*

Social Studies

Do you wear a uniform to school? The students in the story wore uniforms in the classroom, but they did not wear uniforms at their school picnic. Study the use of uniforms in different cultures and in different institutions. Which schools in your community require uniforms to be worn in school? (MI = V/L)

Mathematics

The illustrator of the book, Karen Dugan, uses repetition in her art work. In dyads or triads of students, select a picture from the story to study for repetition of people, animals, buildings, food, or other items. Design a chart which categorizes your findings.Write a question for your classmates so they will need to use multiplication skills to determine the answer. (MI = V/S, L/M, V/L, I/S)

Science

Halmoni served kimbap at the picnic in a small dish with soy sauce. What is soy sauce? How is it made? Place a dot of soy sauce on your tongue with a cotton swab (Q-tip). What do you taste? Place the cotton swab on different parts of your tongue.
Study a diagram of a tongue. Why do you taste the soy sauce sometimes and not at other times? Discuss the use of other spices in enhancing the flavor of food. What spices would people use if they were on a low sodium diet for high blood pressure? (MI = V/L, B/K)

Language Arts

Create a list of new vocabulary words in Korean and English from the story. Role play these words with mannerisms and customs as you practice them. Spell the words phonetically on flashcards to help you pronounce the words. (MI = V/L, V/S)

Physical Education

At the picnic, the third graders played soccer and jumped rope. Why are games and sports often played at picnics? Discuss why you need to balance the food you eat with physical activity to maintain or improve your weight. Name physical activities that you like to do at a picnic. Choose one or two of these activities to do during recess or physical education class this week. (MI = B/K, V/L)

Art

Observe the different borders around each picture in the book. Name different cultures that tend to use borders for their artistic work. What kinds of artistic works have borders? What can be said about perspectives of angles and levels after viewing the beautiful pictures in the book? (MI = V/S, V/L)

Music

Jump rope rhymes have been very popular over the years. Study the rhythm of the jump rope chant in the story or any of the chants found in the book called *Anna Banana and Other Jump Rope Rhymes* (Cole, 1993). See the Teaching Resources at the end of this book. Write your own chant and practice saying it as you jump rope. Encourage your friends to clap along to help emphasize the change in tempo, volume, or rhythm. (MI = M/R, B/K, I/S)

Across the Curriculum

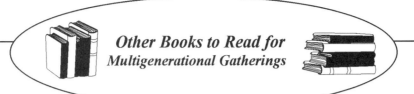

Other Books to Read for
Multigenerational Gatherings

This list contains excellent books to read for learning about Multigenerational Gatherings. Use these books along with the Featured Books when teaching the lessons on the previous pages.

Adams, J. (1991). Going for oysters. Morton Grove, IL: Albert Whitman & Company.
    An Australian girl tells how she fishes for oysters and fish. It is a long and dangerous job. The whole family enjoys eating the fish that she catches.

Aliki. (1979). The two of them. New York: William Morrow & Co., Inc.
    A little girl spends time with her grandfather. They go shopping for food, share a meal together and grow fruit in the garden. An apple tree becomes a good way for the girl to remember her grandfather forever.

Bond, R. (1988). Cherry tree. Honesdale, PA: Boyds Hill Press.
    A young girl from India plants a cherry seed with her grandfather. They observe the tree as it grows through the seasons and eventually it grows quite large. The tree serves as a constant reminder of the girl's grandfather.

dePaola, T. (1993). Tom. New York: Scholastic Inc.
    Tommy has a grandpa who is a butcher that he calls Tom. They spend a lot of time together. Tom gives Tommy some chicken legs, which get him in trouble when he scares a girl at school.

dePaola, T. (1974). Watch out for the chicken feet in your soup. New York: Simon & Schuster Trade.
    Joey and Eugene go to visit Joey's grandma. She feeds them a lot of food and they bake together.

Drucker, M. (1992). Grandma's latkes. San Diego: Harcourt Brace & Co.
    Molly tries to beat her grandmother at grating potatoes, but her grandma is too fast. As Molly and her grandmother make latkes for Hanukkah, her grandmother tells a story about why they celebrate Hanukkah.

Gilman, P. (1990). Grandma and the pirates. New York: Scholastic Inc.
    Grandma, her granddaughter, and a parrot are kidnapped by pirates and taken hostage aboard a ship. The three captives trick the pirates by telling them of hidden treasures. When the pirates get off the ship to search for the treasures, the captives sail away at last.

Other Books to Read,
Continued

Hest, A. (1994). The midnight eaters. New York: Macmillan Children's Book Group.
It's midnight but Sam and her grandmother are still awake and ready for a snack. They sneak downstairs and make ice cream sundaes to eat. They look through old picture albums during their midnight snack.

Hudson, W. (1993). I love my family. New York: Scholastic Inc.
A family takes a summer trip to Grandpa Lawrence's farm in North Carolina. The family enjoys laughing, talking, playing basketball, dancing and having a picnic together. Everyone hates to leave at the end of the week.

Luenn, N. (1990). Nessa's fish. New York: Scholastic Inc.
Nessa and her grandmother catch enough fish to feed the whole camp. However, during the night, Nessa's grandmother becomes sick and Nessa must protect her and the fish from wild animals.

McDonald, M. (1991). A great pumpkin switch. New York: Orchard Books.
Grandpa tells the story of making apple butter when he was a little boy. He used a saw that he wasn't allowed to use and destroyed his sister's prize pumpkin. He eventually bought another large pumpkin so his sister never found out.

McDonald, M. (1994). The potato man. New York: Orchard Books.
Grandpa tells a story about how he once stole potatoes from a half-blind potato seller. The potato man got him in trouble three times, but grandpa learned to respect the old man and eventually becomes his customer.

McKissack, P. C. (1992). A million fish... more or less. New York: Knopf Books for Young Readers.
Hugh Thomas listens to an adventurous tale from Papa-Daddy and Elder Abbajon about Bayou Clapateaux where exaggerated adventures are thought to happen. Hugh Thomas then embarks on his own fishing trip in Bayou Clapteaux. After catching a million fish, he encounters many animals on the way home. The various animals end up eating his fish and leave Hugh Thomas with only three to show his family.

Nerlove, M. (1989). Passover. Niles, IL: Albert Whitman & Company.
It is time for Passover and a father tells his son the tradition of Passover. He explains the different types of food that are eaten and the hunt that occurs after dinner. They then sing songs together.

*Other Books to Read,
Continued*

Palmisciano, D. (1989). Garden partners. New York: Antheneum Books for Young Readers.
    It's spring so it is time to plant the garden. Grandma and her granddaughter plant tomatoes, corn, potatoes, and lettuce. They work in the garden everyday, and soon they have vegetables for their entire family.

Polacco, P. (1993). The bee tree. New York: Philomel Books.
    A little girl is bored with reading. Her grandpa takes her on a chase which leads to a honey tree. The whole town goes with them and enjoys the honey with biscuits and tea. Grandpa uses the chase to teach his granddaughter that adventure, wisdom and knowledge must be pursued and can be found in books just as easily.

Polacco, P. (1990). Thunder cake. New York: Scholastic Inc.
    A little girl visits her grandma in Michigan and experiences a thunderstorm while she is there. She helps her grandma make a cake during the thunder which helps her to overcome her fear of thunder.

Rice, E. (1990). At grammy's house. New York: Greenwillow Books.
    The grandchildren go to grammy's house every Sunday for brunch. Grammy speaks French and she makes a yummy dinner. After dinner, mom and dad come to pick up the kids and take them home.

Stock, C. (1990). Thanksgiving treat. New York: Macmillan Children's Book Group.
    It is time for Thanksgiving and everyone is busy running around to get ready for the big feast. The youngest child wants to help, but everyone tells him he isn't needed. His grandpa comes to the rescue and makes everyone happy.

Tobias, T. (1993). Pot luck. New York: Lothrop, Lee and Shepard Books.
    Rachel and her grandmother prepare for a special dinner guest, Sophie, who is grandmother's oldest friend. They go through a lot of work to make sure everything is perfect.

Van Woerkom, D. (1975). Becky and the bear. New York: G.P. Putnam's Sons.
    Becky's father and brother go hunting for some food while she stays at home with Granny. Becky wishes she was old enough to go hunting and be brave. When Granny has to leave, Becky is left behind to finish some chores and is chased by a large bear.

Weston, M. (1994). Apple juice tea. New York: Houghton Mifflin Company.
    When Gran first comes to visit, Polly wishes she would leave so her life could get back to normal. One night, Gran babysits and they have a tea party. After that, there are many more tea parties and special times.

Focused Theme:
Multicultural Connections

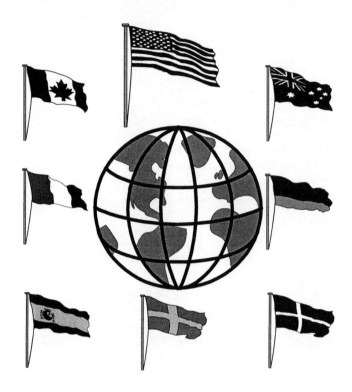

Overview of Multicultural Connections

This focused theme explores concepts of diversity and culture in the context of food and nutrition. Some similarities and differences surface when we compare how we eat, when we eat, and with whom we eat during celebrations, holidays, and everyday meals. Several featured books show what it's like to prepare and enjoy food with our family and friends of different backgrounds and heritages.

Featured Book #1
of the Focused Theme:
Multicultural Connections

Knoxville, Tennessee
by Nikki Giovanni
Scholastic Inc., 1994

This lesson addresses the following Dietary Guidelines for Americans:
⇒ *1. Eat a variety of foods.*
⇒ *2. Balance the food you eat with physical activity; maintain or improve your weight.*
⇒ *3. Choose a diet with plenty of grain products, vegetables, and fruits.*
   4. Choose a diet low in fat, saturated fat, and cholesterol.
   5. Choose a diet moderate in sugars.
   6. Choose a diet moderate in salt and sodium.
   7. Choose an alcohol and drug-free lifestyle.

This lesson highlights the following food groups from the Food Guide Pyramid:
⇒ *Bread, Cereal, Rice, & Pasta Group*
   Fruit Group
⇒ *Vegetable Group*
⇒ *Milk, Yogurt, & Cheese Group*
⇒ *Meat, Poultry, Fish, Dry Beans, Eggs, & Nuts Group*

Food Guide Pyramid
A Guide to Daily Food Choices

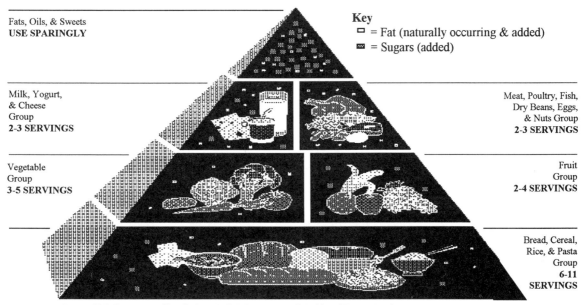

Source: U.S. Department of Agriculture & U.S. Department of Health and Human Services

Lesson Plans for Featured Book 1

Giovanni, N. (1994). <u>Knoxville, tennessee</u>. New York: Scholastic, Inc.
A young girl likes summer best because of the fresh corn from her daddy's garden; the okra, barbecue; and homemade ice cream from the church picnic; and the gospel music from the church homecoming. She also likes to go the mountains with her grandmother where she feels safe and warm. Beginning reading level.

Pre-Reading Activities for *Knoxville, Tennessee*

Have you ever traveled or visited Knoxville, Tennessee? Use a map to determine the number of miles and kilometers between your town and Knoxville. How many states would you drive through if traveling by car or bus? What roads would you take to get to Knoxville? How long would it take in hours? In minutes? Compare the costs in time and money for traveling by car, bus, train, or plane. (MI = V/S, L/M)

Write the Chamber of Commerce in Knoxville or visit a travel agency to plan a hypothetical trip to Knoxville. What travel literature can you preview before your trip? (MI = V/L, B/K)

Post-Reading Activities for *Knoxville, Tennessee*

Questions to develop thinking skills (Bloom's Taxonomy)

1. Knowledge:	Write a list of all the reasons why this girl loves summer the best.
2. Comprehension:	Explain why Knoxville, Tennessee is not mentioned in the story. Recognize that the story might also be told in another city or regional area of the United States.
3. Application:	Report on one of your favorite summer activities.
4. Analysis:	Compare the activities you love to do in the summer to the activities this girl loved. List the similarities and the differences.
5. Synthesis:	Create a poem about eating at a picnic during the summer.
6. Evaluation:	Define or discuss whether this girl has a "healthy" lifestyle. Give examples from the pictures in the book.

Solo Work for *Knoxville, Tennessee*

List all the different picnics you have attended in your lifetime. Talk to your parents or guardians so they can help you remember. Give a name to each of the picnics. What do the names tell you about the focus of the celebration? (MI = I/I, V/L)

Small Group Work for *Knoxville, Tennessee*

Discuss the different dimensions of health. Personal health includes physical health, social health, emotional health, and intellectual (mental) health. Give some examples of physical health from pictures in the book. Place the different foods from the story into the food pyramid. Are there other examples of physical health besides food? Give examples of social health and emotional health from the book too. Are there other dimensions of health that we haven't mentioned from the story? (MI = V/S, I/S)

Whole Class Work for *Knoxville, Tennessee*

In the story, a blanket or quilt is used for a picnic on the ground and for a covering on the bed. Create a paper patchwork quilt using an 8" x 10" or 9" x 12" piece of paper. Use a ruler to draw a triangle in the center of each piece of paper so that students have a border for their artistic work. The triangles also add an overall connecting pattern to the entire quilt when it is assembled. Cut the edges of the quilt squares with pinking shears before attaching it on colorful bulletin board paper or a piece of fabric. Students should work on individual quilt blocks, representing the physical, social, emotional, and intellectual (mental) dimensions of their health. Give a title to the large class quilt then display it in the hallway outside your classroom or in the cafeteria. (MI = V/S, L/M, B/K)

Across the Curriculum for *Knoxville, Tennessee*

Social Studies

Why is there often food when people come together for a celebration, a meeting, or an activity? Discuss some of the ways that people use food in physical, social, emotional, and intellectual (mental) ways. (MI = V/L)

Mathematics

Using a ruler, yardstick, and a tape measure, determine how large your classroom quilt will be based on the number of quilt blocks. If every person makes four quilt blocks for the quilt, how big will the quilt be? Decide if you want your quilt to be rectangular or square. If you hypothetically planned to use your quilt for a picnic blanket, how many people would be able to fit onto it? What would be enough sitting space for an adult? A child? (MI = L/M)

Science

Do you like picnics? Most people love to take a blanket and sit outside to eat. You can feel the sun on your face and watch the ants march toward your lunchbox. Investigate the sense of odor and movement on the food-gathering habits of animals. Ants are not the only "bugs" marching toward to your food to eat it. Foods are very good hosts to microorganisms called *staphacocci aureus*. These bacteria start to multiply quickly when cold food is not kept cold and hot food is not kept hot. The human nose and taste buds can not accurately detect the presence of these organisms. After we consume them we become very sick with vomiting, diarrhea, and headaches. Study a way that heat conduction can be minimized at a picnic. While you are at it, study the effects of radiation on your skin, the effects of convection at a food grill, and the role of convection when it's hot outside. Enjoy the picnic, but don't feed the ants. (MI = V/L)

Language Arts

Write five descriptive sentences about running barefoot across different surfaces. How about a grassy meadow, sandy beach, hot sidewalk, and a stone driveway? What will be your fifth surface? (MI = V/L)

Physical Education

At a class picnic or during recess, encourage students to jump rope. Jump with feet together, using one rotation of the rope for each jump. Also try running in place with high knees, or jumping on one foot while turning the rope. Remember to turn the rope with your wrists and forearms and not by moving your arms in big circles. Jump when the rope moves toward your feet. Skills developed: cardiovascular endurance, jumping, rhythm, and coordination. (MI = B/K, M/R)

Art

Study the effects of mood on art. The illustrator, Larry Johnson, uses combinations of blues and greens to set the tone for Knoxville, Tennessee. Discuss the effects of yellow, white, and red against this background. (MI = V/S)

Music

Gospel music is an integral part of African American culture. Select and sing some of these songs in class. (MI = M/R, V/L)

Across the Curriculum

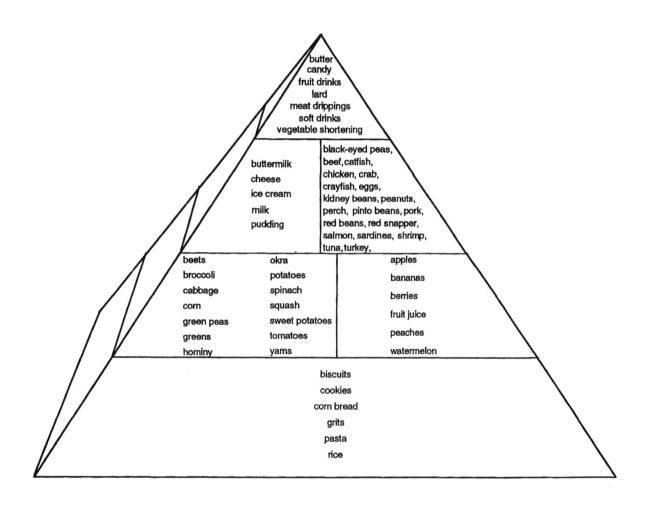

**African American Foods
and the Food Guide Pyramid**

Source: 1993 *Pyramid Packet*, Penn State Nutrition Center,
5 Henderson Building, University Park, PA 16802; (814) 865-6323.

*Featured Book #2
of the Focused Theme:
Multicultural
Connections*

Too Many Tamales
by Gary Soto and Ed Martinez
The Putnam & Grosset Group,
1993

This lesson addresses the following Dietary Guidelines for Americans:
1. Eat a variety of foods.
2. Balance the food you eat with physical activity; maintain or improve your weight.
⇒ 3. *Choose a diet with plenty of grain products, vegetables, and fruits.*
4. Choose a diet low in fat, saturated fat, and cholesterol.
5. Choose a diet moderate in sugars.
6. Choose a diet moderate in salt and sodium.
7. Choose an alcohol and drug-free lifestyle.

This lesson highlights the following food groups from the Food Guide Pyramid:
⇒ *Bread, Cereal, Rice, & Pasta Group*
Fruit Group
Vegetable Group
Milk, Yogurt, & Cheese Group
⇒ *Meat, Poultry, Fish, Dry Beans, Eggs, & Nuts Group*

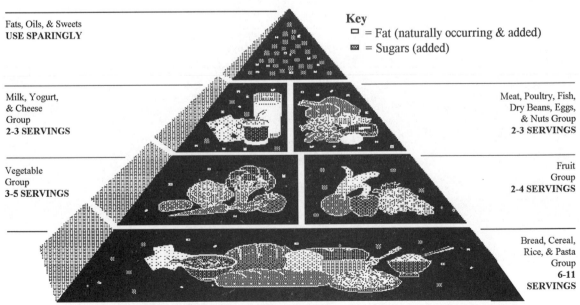

Food Guide Pyramid
A Guide to Daily Food Choices

Fats, Oils, & Sweets
USE SPARINGLY

Key
◻ = Fat (naturally occurring & added)
▨ = Sugars (added)

Milk, Yogurt,
& Cheese
Group
2-3 SERVINGS

Meat, Poultry, Fish,
Dry Beans, Eggs,
& Nuts Group
2-3 SERVINGS

Vegetable
Group
3-5 SERVINGS

Fruit
Group
2-4 SERVINGS

Bread, Cereal,
Rice, & Pasta
Group
**6-11
SERVINGS**

Source: U.S. Department of Agriculture & U.S. Department of Health and Human Services

Lesson Plans for Featured Book 2

Soto, G., & Martinez, E. (1993). Too many tamales. New York: Putnam Publishing Group.
Maria is excited because it is Christmas Eve and she is helping her family make tamales for the holiday. When Maria's mom leaves the kitchen, Maria tries on her mom's ring. Maria thinks she loses the ring in the tamale mix and tries to find it. Intermediate reading level.

Pre-Reading Activities for *Too Many Tamales*

Think about a time when you lost something and could not find it. How did you feel? What problem solving steps did you use to try and find the item? Were your efforts successful? (MI = I/I)

What activities at home make you feel grown up? In what ways, do you act responsibly at home? For example, describe at least one chore you do at home each day. (MI = V/L)

Post-Reading Activities for *Too Many Tamales*

Questions to develop thinking skills (Bloom's Taxonomy)

1. Knowledge: Tell what Maria lost while making tamales.

2. Comprehension: Explain the order of events that led to her problem in this story.

3. Application: Report the events of the evening the way Maria might write the story.

4. Analysis: Observe the way Maria's family prepared the tamales. Do you think they washed their hands first? Why is it important to wash your hands before preparing any food?

5. Synthesis: Improve the way the children set out to find the ring by giving different solutions to their problem.

6. Evaluation: Recommend various side dishes to go with the main dish of tamales. Decide if your recommendations create a well-balanced meal according to the Food Guide Pyramid.

Solo Work for *Too Many Tamales*

Use a paper plate to design and color a festive dish similar to those shown in the book. Use another paper plate to draw the design from the plates you eat on at home. (MI = V/S, B/K)

Small Group Work for *Too Many Tamales*

From a newspaper or magazine, cut out pictures of toys and foods that you most enjoy playing during different holidays. Categorize the foods into the food guide pyramid hung on a bulliten board. Place your toys into the categories of action toys or quiet toys. (MI = V/S, B/K, L/M)

Whole Class Work for *Too Many Tamales*

Using the Food Guide Pyramid as your guide, plan a festive Mexican-American meal. Will it be a Mexican-American meal for breakfast, lunch, or dinner? How many different food groups will you use in your meal? Mexican-American food is a good example of how foods can be combined to make a combination food. Combination foods consists of a variety of foods from different food groups on the Food Guide Pyramid. For example, a burrito contains a tortilla, cheese, and meat or beans. What will you drink with your meal? Maybe you can select a fruit juice, vegetable juice, or water to create a complete combination meal!

Have you ever compared traditional Mexican-American restaurants and fast food Mexican-American restaurants? What are some similarities and differences between the two? Make a list of foods from each type of restaurant using both Spanish and English words. How many combination foods are there on your lists?

If all this talk of food makes you hungry, make some tamales! Working in small groups, mix enough dough for the tamales like they did in the story. Place the dough into a corn shuck, then add a meat or bean mixture in the center. Put some more dough over the top before you fold the corn shuck over the mixture. Tie the shucks closed with a string. Steam the tamales and enjoy as a meal! (MI = V/L, L/M, B/K, I/S)

Across the Curriculum for *Too Many Tamales*

Social Studies

Research the history of different festivals in the Hispanic culture. How do these compare to your own? (MI = V/L)

Mathematics

Count the number of students and teachers in your class. If each person ate 2 tamales, how many would be needed? If each person only ate one-half of a tamale, how many would be needed? (MI = L/M)

Science

In the story, the children ate too many tamales. Did you ever eat too much food? Do you remember what you felt like? When your stomach is too full, it sends out signals that you are bloated and nauseated. Your stomach will push the food into your small intestine, then later you may experience diarrhea, because the food was not adequately digested. Overeating in this way is not healthy nor does it make you feel good. In the story, the children were afraid that one of them had swallowed the diamond ring. Sometimes small children will put objects into their mouths that are inappropriate like a button or a dime. This is very dangerous, because it can block the air passages in the throat. If the object is swallowed and goes into the stomach, it may need to be X-rayed by a physician. If the object is small enough, with no sharp edges and not harmful, it will travel through the intestines and exit the body as a waste product. The individual may experience gut pain and diarrhea. If the object is too large or too sharp, the doctor must perform surgery to remove the object. It's best not to eat non-food items and not to overeat -- even your favorite foods. So enjoy two or three tamalas not 10 or 12! (MI = V/L)

Language Arts

Write a report on the different ways people celebrate a holiday. In the book they are celebrating Christmas. How do other cultures celebrate Christmas? What holidays and festival foods are celebrated by other ethnic groups? (MI = V/L)

Physical Education

Create your own version of the Mexican Hat Dance by using locomotor skills like galloping, sliding, and walking. Also use non-locomotor skills iike bending, twisting, swaying, and clapping. Be able to demonstrate your dance to your guests and other classes during your festival meal. (Skills developed: locomotor and non-locomotor skills). (MI = B/K, M/R)

Art

Read the copyright page in the front of the book. Notice it states that "The text is set in Berkeley Oldstyle." What does this mean? Do other books have this information? What different lettering can you create on a computer to make a menu for your class festival? Or does anyone know what calligraphy is? (MI = V/S, V/L)

Music

Perform a variety of clapping and stomping rhythms when listening to Hispanic music during your festival. Later you can listen to siesta music during a quiet time in class. What tempo of music do you prefer? (MI = M/R)

Across the Curriculum

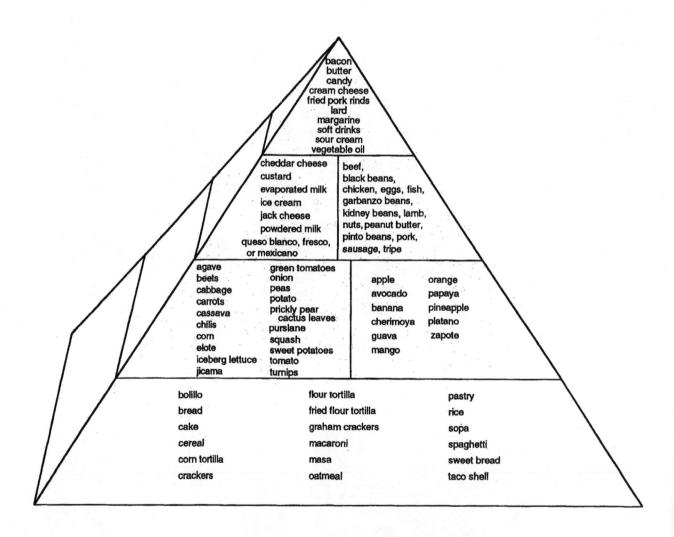

Mexican American Foods
and the Food Guide Pyramid

Source: 1993 *Pyramid Packet*, Penn State Nutrition Center,
5 Henderson Building, University Park, PA 16802; (814) 865-6323.

Featured Book #3 of the Focused Theme: Multicultural Connections

The Relatives Came
by Cynthia Rylant
Macmillan Children's Book Group, 1993

This lesson addresses the following Dietary Guidelines for Americans:

⇒ *1. Eat a variety of foods.*
    2. Balance the food you eat with physical activity; maintain or improve your weight.
⇒ *3. Choose a diet with plenty of grain products, vegetables, and fruits.*
⇒ *4. Choose a diet low in fat, saturated fat, and cholesterol.*
⇒ *5. Choose a diet moderate in sugars.*
    6. Choose a diet moderate in salt and sodium.
    7. Choose an alcohol and drug-free lifestyle.

This lesson highlights the following food groups from the Food Guide Pyramid:

⇒ *Bread, Cereal, Rice, & Pasta Group*
⇒ *Fruit Group*
    Vegetable Group
    Milk, Yogurt, & Cheese Group
⇒ *Meat, Poultry, Fish, Dry Beans, Eggs, & Nuts Group*

Food Guide Pyramid
A Guide to Daily Food Choices

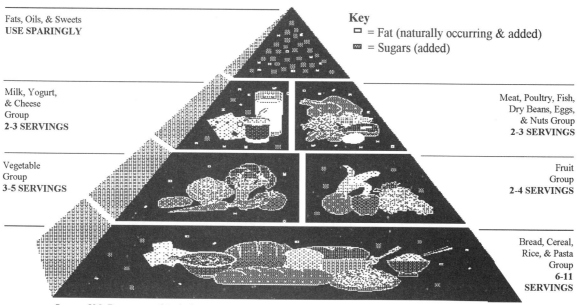

Source: U.S. Department of Agriculture & U.S. Department of Health and Human Services

Lesson Plans for Featured Book 3

Rylant, C. (1985). <u>The relatives came.</u> New York: Macmillan Children's Book Group. Relatives visit from Virginia and bring lots of laughter, hugs, food, and good times. During the reunion, they eat, sleep, and breathe together. Intermediate reading level.

Pre-Reading Activities for *The Relatives Came*

Describe an occasion when you spent an entire day and evening with your relatives. What do you remember most about your time together? (MI = I/I, V/L)

Talk about the regional differences in food and meal-related words. Who drinks pop? Who drinks soda pop? Who drinks soda? Who drinks cola? Who eats dinner? Who eats supper? Can you think of other words with regional overtones? (MI = V/L)

Post-Reading Activities for *The Relatives Came*

<u>Questions to develop thinking skills</u> (Bloom's Taxonomy)

1. Knowledge: From what part of the United States did the relatives come?

2. Comprehension: Discuss the type of celebration that brought the relatives together. How often do these celebrations occur?

3. Application: Pretend you have relatives visiting. Knowing that they have just driven for a very long time to get to your home, fix them a nutritious, well-balanced meal. List the foods you would serve.

4. Analysis: Compare the different foods the relatives eat enroute to the family gathering with the foods they eat upon their arrival. What foods are lowest in fat, saturated fat, and cholesterol? Categorize the different foods into the five food groups.

5. Synthesis: What if the people in the book drove to visit their relatives in Virginia instead? How would the trip and food be different?

6. Evaluation: Consider the time it takes to pack and unpack for a road trip. Judge how long the preparation took for the relatives who came from Virginia as compared to the relatives who came from town.

Solo Work for *The Relatives Came*

When you eat a food at home during this week, empty and clean out the container or wrapper and bring it into class for use. (MI = B/K)

Small Group Work for *The Relatives Came*

Organize a hypothetical six-hour trip by car to visit your relatives. You have space in your car to take one cooler for fresh foods and a milk crate for dry goods. Make a list of foods and beverages you plan to take. Use the empty food containers and wrappers that your class collected during the week to load in the cooler and milk crate. How well can you pack food for your trip? (MI = V/L, I/S, B/K, V/S)

Whole Class Work for *The Relatives Came*

Once you arrive at your hypothetical destination by small groups, unpack your coolers and milk crates to determine the nutrient values of your meals. For example, study food labels to determine the following fun contests:

1) How many foods did you bring from each food group? Which group has the most food from the bread group? Vegetable group? Fruit group? Milk group? and Meat group?

2) How many beverages did you bring? Were your selections only from the milk group? How many beverages were high in sugar? Were any beverages high in sodium? Did you remember to bring water?

3) After sorting your foods for *lunch*, study the food labels to see what your daily values are for one serving of **each** of the food groups. Do your daily values total 100%? How much are they under 100% or over 100%? What do daily values mean?

4) After sorting your foods for *dinner*, find the food which has the highest grams of fat per serving. Which one has the lowest grams of fat per serving? Which food has the lowest milligrams of sodium per serving? Which one has the lowest milligrams of sodium per serving?

5) What foods did you bring for snacks on your trip? Among all the small groups in your class, determine who brought similar packaged snacks. Popcorn? Chips? Crackers? Cookies? Candy? Take one type of food like chips and have a student from each small group bring the food to the front of the class to hold. Have the students order themselves in a human graph from left to right from least fat per serving to most fat per serving. Repeat for sodium. Some foods like cookies and candy can be studied for their sugar content as well as their fat content. Finally, as a whole class make a list of some alternative choices for healthful snacks on roadtrips or anytime!

6) Finish your Food Label Exploration trip by eating one of the most healthful snacks around — cereal! Read different food labels to see why! How many groups remembered to pack cereal? (MI = V/L, L/M, V/S)

Across the Curriculum for *The Relatives Came*

Social Studies

How do myths, sayings, and old wive's tales originate? Determine if there is any truth to some of these sayings: Early to bed, early to rise, makes a person healthy, wealthy, and wise; Eat breakfast like a king, lunch like a prince, and dinner like a peasant; Eat the crusts of your bread so your hair will get nice and curly.
(MI = V/L, L/M)

Mathematics

A person needs at least eight cups of water daily. How many ounces are in one cup of water? How many ounces are in eight cups of water? There are not any substitutes for water. Not pop. Not lemonaide. Not juice. Sure those drinks contain fluids, but your kidneys will also need to use water to break down the sugar in the drink. So drink your water! Do you know how many teaspoons of sugar are in one can of pop?
(MI = L/M)

Science

Determine how long the relatives stayed for their visit by observing the moon in the story. How long does a full moon last? How many days are there between full moons? What else do you know about the moon? (MI = V/L, L/M)

Language Arts

Preparation for bedtime usually requires a regular routine of daily habits. A consistent plan that becomes automatic over time can help you fall asleep faster. Write a sequence story with pictures showing the steps you take to get ready for bed.
(MI = V/L)

Physical Education

Suitcases can be quite heavy and awkward to carry. Load several suitcases with clothing, shoes, and supplies and lift them several times while in a stationary position. Next lift and carry the suitcases for a distance. Who can lift the different weighted bags into an imaginary car? Talk with your physical education teacher about the proper techniques for lifting so you can prevent injuries to your back, arms, and legs.
(MI = B/K)

Art

The illustrator, Stephen Gammell, uses colored pencils to draw the pictures in the book, *The Relatives Came.* Draw a low-fat food and a high-fat food using colored pencils. Where does the food fit on the Food Guide Pyramid? (MI = V/S)

Music

Listen to Appalachian music and try to hear the different instruments making the music. Can you hear the hammered dulcimer, banjo, the autoharp, the fiddle, the bass, the guitar, or the zither? What instruments are shown in the book? (MI = M/R, V/S)

Across the Curriculum

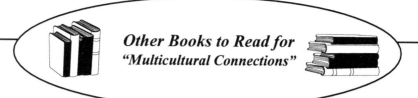

Other Books to Read for
"Multicultural Connections"

This list contains excellent books to read for learning about Multicultural Connections. Use these books along with the Featured Books when teaching the lessons on the previous pages.

Adoff, A. (1971). Ma nda la. New York: HarperCollins Children's Books.
    Pictures and the words Ra, Ma, La and Ha tell a story of a boy and his parents who plant corn, weed it, watch it grow, harvest it, then eat it.

Aylesworth, J. (1992). The folks in the valley. New York: HarperCollins Children's Books.
    Using the Pennsylvania Dutch culture as a backdrop, this book uses a rhyme to teach the alphabet. For example, the letter "E" is represented by the rhyme "Eggs are found under the fat red hens."

Bang, M. (1984). The grey lady and the strawberry snatcher. New York: Macmillan Children's Books.
    A man with a passion for strawberries gives an old lady some strawberries to take home. On her way home, the strawberry snatcher tries to steal her strawberries. After failed attempts, the strawberry snatcher settles on eating blackberries from a nearby bush. (Wordless book).

Bider, D. (1989). A drop of honey. New York: Simon & Schuster Books for Young Readers.
    Anayida falls asleep and dreams of baking baklava. When she buys the honey, she drops some of it on the sidewalk. A bee lands on the honey and a cat chases the bee. A dog chases the cat and they all run through the town. The whole town is turned upside down because of one drop of honey.

Cohen, B. (1987). The carp in the bathtub. Rockville, MD: Kar-Ben Copies, Inc.
    Leah and Henry want to save the carp that their mom will want to cook for dinner. They try to hide the carp in the tub and also in a bucket. Their dad explains that fish are for eating so he gives them a cat as a pet.

Falwell, C. (1993). Feast for 10. New York: Scholastic Inc.
    A family goes shopping. As they find the groceries, they count each item as it is put in the cart. When they get home, they unload the groceries and count the items as they take them out.

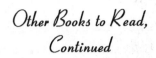

Other Books to Read,
Continued

Freidman, I. R. (1984). <u>How my parents learned to eat</u>. Boston: Houghton Mifflin Co.
   A little girl tells the story of how her mother and father met. Her father was a sailor and he met his future wife in Japan. She teaches him how to eat with chopsticks and he teaches her how to eat with silverware.

Goldin, B. D. (1993). <u>Cakes and miracles: A purim tale</u>. New York: Puffin Books.
   Hershel is a blind boy who loves to play outside and catch frogs in the river. His mother is always angry when he comes home covered with mud. One day Hershel has a dream that he can see. After that, he is able to help his mom make three-cornered fat cakes and cookies to sell at the market so they can earn money.

Goldin, B. D. (1988). <u>Just enough is plenty: A hanukkah tale</u>. New York: Puffin Books.
   It is almost time for Hanukkah. Malka's family invites a peddler for dinner. They are surprised when they wake up in the morning and find that the peddler has left behind wonderful gifts.

Howard, E. F. (1991). <u>Aunt flossie's hat (and crab cakes later)</u>. New York: Dell Publishers Co, Inc.
   Susan and Sarah spend a Sunday afternoon with their Aunt Flossie. As they try on her old hats, Aunt Flossie tells a story associated with each one. Afterwards, they celebrate with their favorite food-crab cakes.

Kroll, S. (1989). <u>The hokey-pokey man</u>. New York: Holiday House Inc.
   Ben and Sarah, two children in New York City in the early 20th century, are friends with Joe, the ice cream man. With the help of his cousin, Joe surprises the city with a new concept of ice cream cones. The children almost ruin his surprise.

Lessac, F. (1989). <u>Caribbean alphabet</u>. New York: William Morrow & Co., Inc.
   Through a colored panoramic view of the Caribbean, different items are shown through letters of the alphabet. An example for the letter M is melons.

Manushkin, F. (1992). <u>Latkes and applesauce</u>. New York: Scholastic Inc.
   A snowstorm limits the supply of apples and potatoes during Hanukkah. A family gives shelter to a hungry kitten and a puppy, which deepens the meaning of the holiday.

Manushkin, F. (1995). <u>The matzah that papa brought home</u>. New York: Scholastic Inc.
   A little girl and her family celebrate the Passover Seder in repeating rhyme form. The family feasts on matzah, bitter herbs, green vegetables, and haroset.

Other Books to Read,
Continued

Mitchell, B., & Sandford, J. (1993). <u>Down buttermilk lane</u>. New York: Lothrop, Lee & Shepard.
  An Amish family goes away for a day to buy clothes and food. They return home to eat dinner,
  then take their animals to the barn.

Obligado, L. (1993). <u>The chocolate cow</u>. New York: Simon & Schuster Books for Young Readers.
  Pierre is worried that his father might sell Melody, his cow. Melody can no longer give milk and
  Pierre's father has no need for her. Pierre decides to do all he can for Melody so she will produce
  milk. He feeds her the best food, and she turns into a very special cow.

Olaleye, I. (1994). <u>Bitter bananas</u>. Honesdale, PA: Boyd's Mill Press.
  Yusuf is a boy who lives in a jungle in Africa. His favorite drink is palm sap, and he sells what
  he doesn't drink. A family of baboons begins to steal his sap, so he tries many things to keep the
  baboons away.

Penn, M. (1994). <u>The miracle of the potato latkes</u>. New York: Holiday House Inc.
  Tanta Golda is a Russian woman who makes the most delicious potato latkes in Russia. This
  year, there is only one tiny potato from the harvest. Tanta doesn't know what to do. When a
  begger comes to her door, she feeds him the one potato. The beggar brings her good luck, and
  there are potato latkes for everyone!

Polacco, P. (1988). <u>Rechenka's eggs</u>. New York: Philomel Books.
  Old Babushka is preparing her painted eggs for the Easter Festival. One day she finds a
  wounded goose and takes it back to her house. As the goose recovers, it accidentally knocks
  over the basket of painted eggs. Rechenka pays Babushka back by laying eggs that win in the
  Easter Festival.

Priceman, M. (1994). <u>How to make an apple pie and see the world</u>.   New York: Knopf Books
  A girl decides to make an apple pie. She goes to the store and finds it closed. Now she must
  travel across the world to gather ingredients for her pie. She goes to Italy, France, Sri Lanka,
  England, Jamaica, and Vermont. Once her ingredients are gathered she takes them home and
  bakes an apple pie.

Other Books to Read,
Continued

Rose, A. (1973). How does a czar eat potatoes? New York: Lothrop, Lee and Shepard Books.
  The life of a peasant farmer and the czar are compared and contrasted by the peasant's child.

Steffy, J. (1987). The school picnic. Intercourse, PA: Good Books.
  Amish children have a full day of activities which start very early in the morning. After school,
  all the children and their parents go on a large picnic and have lots of fun.
  them. A clever market lady tries to gather all the mangos so she can sell them.

Valens, A. (1993). Danilo the fruitman. New York: Dial Books For Young Readers.
  Danilo, the fruitman, sells oranges to all the people in town. One day he discovers a new fruit,
  but when he tries to sell it, people just laugh at him. When he discovers the secret of this fruit,
  he becomes very popular with all the people.

Watson, P., & Watson, M. (1994). The market lady and the mango tree. New York: Wm. Morrow.
  The children in the village see many things they want to buy. However, they have no money, so
  they must wait until the mangos fall off the trees. Once mangos have fallen, anyone can eat.

Williams, S. A. (1992). Working cotton. New York: Harcourt Brace & Co.
  Shelan's family arrives in the field along with many other people to harvest the cotton. Shelan
  watches her mom, dad, and sisters picking cotton and she wishes she could pick it as fast as they
  can. Everyone works hard, breaking only for lunch of cornbread and greens.

Williams, V. B. (1991). Cherries and cherry pits. New York: Scholastic Inc.
  A girl and her friend make up stories to go with the pictures she draws. All the stories have to do
  with eating cherries.

Zimelman, N. (1976). I will tell you of peach stone. New York: Lothrop, Lee, and Shepard Books.
  A wise old man and his dog bring the gift of the peach from China to the rest of the world.

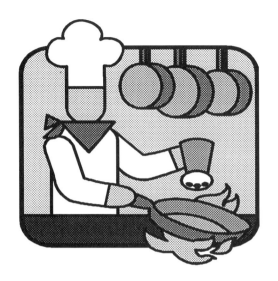

Letter to Food Service Professionals

Our class is studying a nutrition and health unit called "World of People". We will study the diversity of people from a cultural and aging perspective while exploring the different foods that they eat and enjoy. When your schedule permits, would you be willing to team with us to help us learn? We would like to use your cafeteria facilities and some of your equipment during a few of our lessons. For example, we may need to use several of your lunchroom trays, your refrigerator, a large mixing bowl, mixing spoons, and large pots for boiling dumplings. We would also like to use the heating element and a pot to boil the eggs (or an egg cooker for hard boiling the eggs). On our festival day, we would like to decorate some of the cafeteria tables to use during our meal. We will also need the cafeteria one afternoon for a fashion show, egg auction, and afternoon tea.

Thank you for helping us to learn!

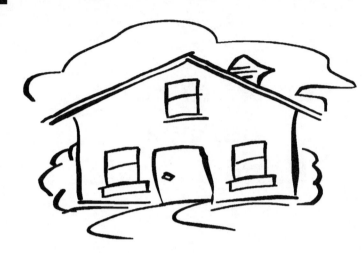

Letter to Parents and Caregivers

We are starting our final nutrition and health unit called "World of People". We will learn about the world of diversity within our families and outside our family unit as it relates to food, nutrition, and health. In order to have the best possible learning experience in this unit, would you please contribute one of the needed items below? Anything you can do to help us by _____(date) will be greatly appreciated. We would also like you to join us in class on _____(date).

- 1 package of egg roll wrappers
- 1 box of wax paper
- 1 sack of oranges, bananas, apples, pears, or other fruit in season
- 1 can of pineapple
- colorful toothpicks
- 1 box of instant rice (or rice to be steamed in a rice cooker)
- 1 jar of honey
- 1 package of bok choy, cabbage, onions, celery, cooked chicken
- 1 pie crust mix
- 1 package of popsickle sticks
- 6 hard cooked (boiled) eggs in the carton
- 1 bag of plaster of paris
- 1 package of balloons
- scraps of ribbons, feathers, lace, fabric or other craft items suitable to trim and decorate hats
- 1 bolt of ribbon
- cardboard tubes
- construction paper
- 1 bottle of soy sauce
- 1 box of cotton swabs (Q-tips)
- tape measure

Thank you kindly!

For the Pleasure of Reading

This booklist can be sent home during Unit 5: World of People, so that your students and their families can read additional literature about food and nutrition together. You can also place these books in your classroom library during the unit. These books are considered secondary resources for this unit. Each book and its abstract is listed as a primary resource in another unit. Use the index at the back of this book to see how titles are crosslisted with other units. Our goal is to show how each book can be used in multiple ways to teach nutrition and health concepts.

Multigenerational Gatherings
Creedle, E. (1934). Down down the mountain. New York: Elscuier/Nelson Books.
Falwell, C. (1993). Feast for 10. New York: Scholastic Inc.
Giovanni, N. (1968). Knoxville, tennessee. New York: Scholastic, Inc.
Joosse, B. M. (1987). Jam day. New York: HarperCollins Children's Books.
Locker, T. (1994). Family farm. New York: Puffin Books.
Manushkin, F. (1995). The matzah that papa brought home. New York: Scholastic Inc.

Multicultural Connections
Adams, J. (1991). Going for oysters. Morton Grove, IL: Albert Whitman & Company.
Agard, J. (1989). The calypso alphabet. New York: Henry Holt & Co., Inc.
Aliki. (1994). Christmas tree memories. New York: HarperCollins Children's Books.
Altman, L. J. (1993). Amelia's road. New York: Lee & Low Books Inc.
Bond, R. (1988). Cherry tree. Honesdale, PA: Boyds Hill Press.
Breinburg, P. (1974). Doctor shawn. New York: Thomas Y. Crowell Company.
Choi, S. N. (1993). Halmoni and the picnic. Boston: Houghton Mifflin Co.
Czernecki, S., & Rhodes, T. (1992). The sleeping bread. New York: Hyperion Paperbacks.
dePaola, T. (1978). The popcorn book. New York: Scholastic Inc.
dePaola, T. (1974). Watch out for the chicken feet in your soup. New York: Simon & Schuster
Falwell, C. (1993). Feast for 10. New York: Scholastic Inc.
Hudson, W. (1993). I love my family. New York: Scholastic Inc.
Lakin, P. (1994). Don't forget. New York: William Morrow & Company Inc.
Luenn, N. (1990). Nessa's fish. New York: Scholastic Inc.
McKissack, P. C. (1992). A million fish... more or less. New York: Knopf Books.
Morris, A. (1989). Bread, bread, bread. New York: Scholastic Inc.
Paulsen, G. (1995). The tortilla factory. San Diego: Harcourt Brace and Co.
Polacco, P. (1993). The bee tree. New York: Philomel Books.
Polacco, P. (1992). Chicken sunday. New York: Scholastic Inc.
Polacco, P. (1990). Thunder cake. New York: Scholastic Inc.
Rattigan, J. K. (1993). Dumpling soup. New York: Little, Brown & Co.
Rice, E. (1990). At grammy's house. New York: Greenwillow Books.
Schaefer, J. J. (1994). Miranda's day to dance. New York: Macmillan Children's Book Group.

References

Achterberg, C., McKenzie, J., & Arosemena, F. (1996). *Multicultural pyramid packet.* University Park, PA: Penn State Nutrition Center.

Armstrong, T. (1994, November). Multiple intelligences: Seven ways to approach curriculum. *Educational Leadership*, 26-28.

Birch, L.L., & Sullivan, S.A. (1991). Measuring children's food preferences. *Journal of School Health, 61(5),* 212-214.

Bloom, B. S. (1956). *Taxonomy of educational objectives. Handbook I: The cognitive domain.* New York: David McKay.

Buscaglia, L. F. (1984). *Loving each other: The challenge of human relationships.* New York: Fawcett Columbine.

Cole, J. (1993). *Anna banana and other jump rope rhymes.* New York: Scholastic Inc.

Erickson, H. L. (1998). *Concept-based curriculum and instruction: Teaching beyond the facts.* Thousand Oaks, CA: Corwin Press, Inc.

Evers, C. L. (1995). *How to teach nutrition to kids: An integrated, creative approach to nutrition education for children ages 6-10.* Tigard, OR: 24 Carrot Press.

Fogarty, R., & Stoeher, J. (1995). *Integrating curricula with multiple intelligences: Team, themes, and threads.* Palatine, IL: IRI/Skylight Training and Publishing, Inc.

Gardner, H. (1983). *Frames of mind: The theory of multiple intelligences.* New York: Basic Books.

Gardner, H. (1995). Reflections on multiple intelligences: Myths and messages. *Phi Delta Kappan*, 77(3), 200-209.

Joint Committee on National Health Education Standards (1995). *National health education standards: Achieving health literacy.* Atlanta, GA: American Cancer Society, Inc.

Krummel, D. A. (1994). National nutrition month and hunger awareness week: A win-win effort. *Journal of the American Dietetic Association*, 94(3), 254-255.

Marx, E., Wooley, S. F., & Northrop, D. (1999). *Health is academic: A guide to coordinated school health programs.* New York: Teachers College Press.

National Research Council (1996). *National science education standards.* National Academy Press: Washington, DC.

Teaching Resources

Food and Nutrition Teaching Manuals and Cookbooks

Albyn, Carole Lisa; Webb, Lois Sinaiko. *The multicultural cookbook for students.* Phoenix, AZ: Oryx Press; 1993; ISBN: 0-89774-735-6.

Bruno, Janet. *Book cooks: Literature-based classroom cooking: 35 recipes for favorite books (Grades K-3).* Cypress, CA; 1991; ISBN: 0-99922-8998-8.

Cobb, Vicki. *Science experiments you can eat.* New York: HarperCollins Publishers; 1994; ISBN: 0-06-023534-9.

Dahl, Felicity. *Roald dahl's revolting recipes.* New York: Scholastic Inc; 1994; ISBN: 0-590-64799-7.

D'Amico, Joan; Drummond, Karen Eich. *The science chef.* New York: John Wiley and Sons; 1995; ISBN: 0-471-31045-X.

Evers, Connie Liakos. *How to teach nutrition to kids: An integrated, creative approach to nutrition education for children ages 6-10.* Tigard, OR: 24 Carrot Press; 1995; ISBN: 0-9647970-3-8.

Feeney, Lisa. *Learning through play: Cooking, A practical guide for teaching young children.* New York: Scholastic Inc; 1992; ISBN: 0-590-49246-2.

Freeman, Darlene. *Cooking projects that make kids think.* Fearon Teacher Aids: Carthage, IL; 1995; ISBN: 0-86653-885-2.

Lief, Patricia. *Fun with fruits and vegetables.* Carthage, IL: Fearon Teacher Aids; 1991; ISBN: 0-86653-994-8.

Ohio Department of Education. *Snackin' smart: Fun activities and recipes your kids will love to eat!* Columbus, OH: Division of Child Nutrition Services, Child and Adult Care Food Program, and the Division of Student Development, Prevention, Health, and Family Involvement, Nutrition Education and Training Program; 1996.

Rothstein, Gloria Lesser. *From soup to nuts.* New York: Scholastic Professional Books; 1994; ISBN: 0-590-49650-6.

Seaman, Rosie. *Food fancies for the young chef.* Fearon Teacher Aids: Carthage, IL; 1995; ISBN: 0-86653-888-7.

Non-Fiction Food and Nutrition Books for Children

Badt, Karin Luisa. *Good morning, let's eat! A world of difference.* Chicago: Childrens Press. ISBN: 0-516-48190-8.

Copsey, Susan Elizabeth. *Children just like me: A unique celebration of children around the world.* New York: Dorling Kindersley (1-800-352-6651); 1995; ISBN: 0-7894-0201-7.

Dibble, Lisa. *The dorling kindersley picturepedia: Food and farming.* New York: Dorling Kindersley; 1993; ISBN: 1-56458-387-2.

Dorling Kindersley. *My little yellow book.* New York: Dorling Kindersley; 1993; ISBN: 1-56458-315-5.

Dorling Kindersley. *My little green book.* New York: Dorling Kindersley; 1993; ISBN: 1-56458-316-3.

Dorling Kindersley. *My little red book.* New York: Dorling Kindersley; 1993; ISBN: 1-56458-313-9.

Dorling Kindersley. *My little brown book.* New York: Dorling Kindersley; 1993; ISBN: 1-56458-318-X.

Dorling Kindersley. *My little orange book.* New York: Dorling Kindersley; 1993; ISBN: 1-56458-314-7.

Dorling Kindersley. *My little blue book.* New York: Dorling Kindersley; 1993; ISBN: 1-56458-317-1.

Evans, David; Williams, Claudette. *Let's explore science: Me and my body.* New York: Dorling Kindersley; 1992; ISBN: 1-56458-121-7.

Parker, Steve. *Eyewitness explorers: Human body -- Investigate and understand your amazing body.* New York: Dorling Kindersley; 1994; ISBN: 1-56458-322-8.

Payne, Fiona. *The dorling kindersley picturepedia: The human body.* New York: Dorling Kindersley; 1993; ISBN: 1-56458-249-3.

Rice, Christopher. *My first body book: With see-through pages to let you look right inside the human body.* New York: Dorling Kindersley; 1995; ISBN: 1-56458-893-9.

Rockwell, Lizzy. *Good enough to eat: A kid's guide to food and nutrition.* New York: HarperCollins; 1999; ISBN: 0-06-027434-4.

Royston, Angela. *What's inside? My body: A first guide to the wonders and workings of the human body.* New York: Dorling Kindersley; 1991; ISBN: 1-879431-07-6.

Showers, Paul. *What happens to a hamburger.* New York: Scholastic Inc; 1985; ISBN 0-590-18911-5.

Smith, Alastair. *What happens to your food?* New York: Scholastic Inc; 1997; ISBN 0-590-97321-5.

Watson, Carol. *My first encyclopedia.* New York: Dorling Kindersley; 1993; ISBN: 1-56458-214-0.

Audiovisual Aids: Cassette Tapes (Songs)

The following music has nutrition and health-related songs for use with our curriculum:

Great American Audio Corp. (1961). *The Little Yellow Learning Bus: Health, Safety, and Feeling Good.*
    Side 1:   Do Not Be a Sugar Junky
                 What to Drink

Beall, Pamela Conn & Nipp, Susan Hagen. (1981). *Wee Sing and Play (including book)*
    Side 1:   Hot Potato (page 9)
                 I Caught a Fish (page 9)
                 Apples, Peaches (page 10)
                 The Seed Cycle (page15)
                 The Muffin Man (page 20)
                 Oats, Peas, Beans (page 32)
    Side 2:   Two Little Sausages (page 37)
                 Who Stole the Cookies from the Cookie Jar? (page 54)
                 Pease Porridge Hot (page 58)

Raffi. (1976). *Singable Songs for the Very Young.*
    Side 1:   I Wonder If I'm Growing
    Side 2:   Peanut Butter Sandwich

Raffi. (1979). *The Corner Grocery Store and other Singable Songs*
    Side 2:   The Corner Grocery Store
                 Popcorn
                 Going on a Picnic

Raffi. (1985). *One Light, One Sun*
    Side 1:   Apples and Bananas
                 In My Garden
    Side 2:   Down on Grandpa's Farm

Raffi. (1994). *Bananaphone.*
    Side 1:   Naturally
    Side 2:   Cowlit Night

Scholastic Inc. (1993). *Thematic Poems, Songs, and Fingerplays (including book)*
    Side 1:   Eat the Alphabet (page 6)
                 The Shape of Things (page 12)
                 The Food to Eat (page 18)

Note: The Raffi and Wee Sing music is available in record, cassette, and compact disc formats from the following vendor: Construction Playthings, 1227 E. 119th Street, Grandview, MO 64030-1117; 1-800-448-4115.

Audiovisual Aids: Cassette Tapes with Picture Books

The following picture books in our curriculum have an accompanying cassette tape available through Scholastic Inc. (1-800-325-6149):

Apples and Pumpkins (Rockwell)
Chicken Soup with Rice (Sedlack)
Feast for 10 (Falwell)
Stone Soup (McGovern)
Growing Vegetable Soup (Rockwell)
This is the Way (Dalton)

Audiovisual Aids: Videotapes

The following vendor has videocassette productions of selected picture books from our curriculum:

Reading Rainbow Videocassettes: Thirty minute programs for 5 to 8 year olds. GPN, University of Nebraska-Lincoln, P.O. Box 80669, Lincoln, NE 68501-0669, (402) 472-2007 or (800) 228-4630.
Videocassettes of selected titles from our curriculum include: Halmoni and the Picnic (Program #106), Rechenka's Eggs (Program #809), Alexander and the Terrible, Horrible, No Good, Very Bad Day (Program #14), Growing Vegetable Soup (Program #100), Cloudy With a Chance of Meatballs (Program #100), The Lady and the Spider (Program #36), Louis the Fish (Program #5), Where the Wild Things Are (Program #5), How My Parents Learned to Eat (Program #18), The Two of Them (Program #22).

Multimedia: CD-ROM

Pyramid Challenge: The CD-ROM Healthy Eating Guide with Curriculum Guide. DINE Systems, Inc., 586 North French Road, Amherst, NY 14228; 1-800-688-1848. Pyramid Challenge is available for IBM Windows and MAC computers, including options for single user, Lab Pack (5 users), and Site License (35 users).

5 A Day Adventures CD-ROM Program was developed by Dole Food Company, Inc. in collaboration with the Society for Nutrition Education. The program is designed to encourage children to eat five servings of fruits and vegetables a day in support of the national "5 A Day For Better Health" Program, sponsored by the National Cancer Institute. The interactive multimedia computer program is free to elementary schools or organizations working directly with children. Send your request on school letterhead and indicate the format and the quantity of CD-ROM discs needed. Allow 4 to 6 weeks for delivery. Mail or Fax your request on school letterhead to: 5 A Day Adventures, Dole Food Company, Inc., 155 Bovet, Suite 476, San Mateo, CA 94402; Fax #: (415) 570-5250.
Note:
A "5 A Day Home Page" is available on the World Wide Web and is accessible at http://www.dole5aday.com
Teachers can e-mail the Dole Teachers Lounge on the Web Site at dole.nutrition@bnt.com
Students can e-mail the 40 fruit and vegetable characters at fiveaday@bev.net

Food and Nutrition Stickers

Mrs. Grossman's Paper Company, 3810 Cypress Drive, Petaluma, CA 94954; 1-800-457-4570. Food stickers.

Mid East United Dairy Industry Association, 5950 Sharon Woods Blvd., Columbus, OH 43220; 614-890-1800; 1-800-292-MILK. Milk, cheese, and ice cream stickers.

Washington State Dairy Council, 4201 - 198th St. S.W. Suite 102, Lynnwood, WA 98036; 206-744-1616; 1-800-470-1222. Pyramid stickers.

Food Pyramid Puzzle

An all wood, 6-piece inlay puzzle of the Food Guide Pyramid is available from the following vendors:

S&S Arts & Crafts: Developmentally Appropriate Materials from Birth to Five, P.O. Box 513, Colchester, CT 06415-0513; 1-800-243-9232.

Construction Playthings, 13201 Arrington Road, Grandview, MO 64030-1117; 1-800-448-4115.

Nasco Hands-On-Health, 901 Janesville Avenue, Fort Atkinson, WI 53538-0901; 1-800-558-9595.

Food Models

Food replicas. Nasco Hands-On-Health, 901 Janesville Avenue, Fort Atkinson, WI 53538-0901; 1-800-558-9595.

Food models for early childhood educators with leader guide. National Dairy Council, 10255 W. Higgins Road, Suite 900, Rosemont, IL 60118-5616; Call 1-800-426-8271 for the Dairy Council nearest you.

Food models: Breakfast food, dinner food #1, dinner food #2, taco treat, asian food, hispanic food, international bread, lunch food, fruits and vegetables, and from the garden. S&S Arts & Crafts: Developmentally Appropriate Materials from Birth to Five, P.O. Box 513, Colchester, CT 06415-0513; 1-800-243-9232.

Food models, market stall, cash register, and shopping cart. Construction Playthings, 13201 Arrington Road, Grandview, MO 64030-1117; 1-800-448-4115.

Food Guide Pyramid Posters (8.5" x 11" tear pad)

Guide to Good Eating and Daily Food Guide Pyramid. National Dairy Council, 10255 W. Higgins Road, Suite 900, Rosemont, IL 60118-5616; Call 1-800-426-8271 for the Dairy Council nearest you.

Food Guide Pyramid Poster. National Live Stock and Meat Board, 444 North Michigan Avenue, Chicago, IL 60611; 312-467-5520; 800-368-3138.

Three-Dimensional Pyramid Model

The pyramid challenge. Rainbow Bread IRONKIDS, P.O. Box 1400K, Dayton, OH 45413-9903

Flannel Boards

Fruits & Vegetables and *Food Pyramid* flannel sets are available from *Construction Playthings,* 13201 Arrington Road, Grandview, MO 64030-1117; 1-800-448-4115.

Classroom Reference Books
Which Include Information on Food and Nutrition

Awesome almanac series of the 50 states: A treasury of facts and fictions, celebrities and celebrations, and the weird and wonderful! Order an almanac about your state from B & B Publishing, Inc., P.O. Box 96, 820 Wisconsin Street, Walworth, WI 53184, or place your order through your local bookstore.

The world almanac for kids 1996. Mahwah, NJ: World Almanac Books; 1995; ISBN: 0-88687-770-9.

Other Nutrition Curricula

The guide to good eating and daily food guide pyramid leader guide. National Dairy Council, 10255 W. Higgins Road, Suite 900, Rosemont, IL 60118-5616; Call 1-800-426-8271 for the Dairy Council nearest you.

Foods around the world. Dairy Council Wisconsin; Call 1-800-993-2479 for a catalog.

Chef combo's fantastic adventures in tasting and nutrition. National Dairy Council, 10255 W. Higgins Road, Suite 900, Rosemont, IL 60118-5616; Call 1-800-426-8271 for the Dairy Council nearest you.

Children's Picture Book Database

The Children's Picture Book Database at Miami University (CPBD@MU) is a bibliography for designing literature-based thematic units for all disciplines, including health education. Find it on the World Wide Web at **http://www.lib.muohio.edu/pictbks**. The database contains abstracts of over 4000 picture books for children, preschool to grade 3. Search over 900 keywords (topics, concepts, and skills) to locate books with storylines adaptable to your curriculum or program. Users can search for book abstracts using a Combination Search (boolean), Alphabetic Search, and/or a Categorical Search. The categories include: Health and Medicine; Social Studies; Natural History and Natural Sciences; Mathematics; Visual and Performing Arts; and Literature, Language and Communication. Content weblinks are also available for many of the keywords, so that users have access to current content information on a topic or concept, and also have a bibliographic listing of children's picture books to teach and learn about the topic, concept, or skill.

Riddles About Different Foods

Bread, Cereal, Rice, & Pasta Group

What do you get when you cross a snowstorm with a cornfield? Cornflakes.

What famous speech did the noodle president give? The Spaghettis-burg Address.

Fruit Group

What fruit do vampires like the best? Neck-tarines.

What goes up in the air green and comes down red? A watermelon.

Vegetable Group

How did the Halloween witch fix her flat bicycle tire? With a pump-kin.

What vegetable is most like a dog? Collie-flower

Milk, Yogurt, & Cheese Group

What happened when Mrs. Moofle found a goat in the refrigerator? It turned to butt-er.

Who grants wishes to unhappy cheeses? The dairy godmother.

Meat, Poultry, Fish, Dry Beans, Eggs, & Nuts Group

When is a turkey most like a ghost? When it's a-goblin'.

What did the octopus have for lunch? A peanut butter and jellyfish sandwich.

Fats, Oils, & Sweets

What kind of cookies do computers like? Chocolate micro-chip.

How do you keep a cookie's jacket closed? With ginger snaps.

Source: Mathews, Judith and Robinson, Fay. (1993). *Oh, how waffle! Riddles you can eat.* Morton Grove, IL: Albert Whitman & Company.

Picture Books Which Include Recipes

Bider, D. (1989). A drop of honey. New York: Simon & Schuster Books for Young Readers.
Darling, B. (1992). Valerie and the silver pear. New York: Macmillan Children's Book Grp.
dePaola, T. (1978). The popcorn book. New York: Scholastic Inc.
dePaola, T. (1974). Watch out for the chicken feet in your soup. New York: Simon & Schuster
Drucker, M. (1992). Grandma's latkes. San Diego: Harcourt Brace & Co.
Goldin, B. D. (1993). Cakes and miracles: A purim tale. New York: Puffin Books.
Lakin, P. (1994). Don't forget. New York: William Morrow & Company Inc.
Manushkin, F. (1992). Latkes and applesause. New York: Scholastic Inc.
McMillan, B. (1991). Eating fractions. New York: Scholastic Inc.
Nottridge, R. (1991). Apples. Minneapolis: Carolrhoda Books, Inc.
Penn, M. (1994). The miracle of the potato latkes. New York: Holiday House Inc.
Polacco, P. (1990). Thunder cake. New York: Scholastic Inc.
Rattigan, J. K. (1993). Dumpling soup. New York: Little, Brown & Co.
Shiefman, V. (1994). Sunday potatoes, monday potatoes. New York: Simon & Schuster
Turner, D. (1989). Bread. Minneapolis: Carolrhoda Books, Inc.
Wagner, K. (1990). Chocolate chip cookies. New York: Henry Holt & Co., Inc.
Wellington, M. (1992). Mr. cookie baker. New York: Dutton Children's Books.

Picture Books Which Offer Content Information through Author Notes

Agard, J. (1989). The calypso alphabet. New York: Henry Holt & Co., Inc.
Altman, L. J. (1993). Amelia's road. New York: Lee & Low Books Inc.
Aylesworth, J. (1992). The folks in the valley. New York: HarperCollins Children's Books.
Christensen, B. (1994). An edible alphabet. New York: Dial Books for Young Readers.
DiSalvo-Ryan, D. (1991). Uncle willie and the soup kitchen. New York: Morrow Junior
Ehlert, L. (1993). Eating the alphabet: Fruits and vegetables from a to z. San Diego: Harcourt Brace & Co.
Forest, H. (1993). The bakers dozen. San Diego: Harcourt Brace & Co.
Goldin, B. D. (1993). Cakes and miracles: A purim tale. New York: Puffin Books.
Goldin, B. D. (1988). Just enough is plenty: A hanukkah tale. New York: Puffin Books.
Kroll, S. (1989). The hokey-pokey man. New York: Holiday House Inc.
Lessac, F. (1989). Caribbean alphabet. New York: William Morrow & Co., Inc.
Manushkin, F. (1992). Latkes and applesause. New York: Scholastic Inc.
Manushkin, F. (1995). The matzah that papa brought home. New York: Scholastic Inc.
McMillan, B. (1991). Eating fractions. New York: Scholastic Inc.
McMillan, B. (1988). Growing colors. New York: Lothrup, Lee and Shepard Books.
Morris, A. (1989). Bread, bread, bread. New York: Scholastic Inc.
Nerlove, M. (1989). Passover. Niles, IL: Albert Whitman & Company.
Obligado, L. (1993). The chocolate cow. New York: Simon & Schuster Books.
Rattigan, J. K. (1993). Dumpling soup. New York: Little, Brown & Co.
Schaefer, J. J. (1994). Miranda's day to dance. New York: Macmillan Children's Book Group.
Valens, A. (1993). Danilo the fruitman. New York: Dial Books For Young Readers.
Williams, S. A. (1992). Working cotton. New York: Harcourt Brace & Co.

Adams, J. (1991). Going for oysters. **Units 5, 2, 3**

Adoff, A. (1971). Ma nda la. **Units 5, 4**

Agard, J. (1989). The calypso alphabet. **Unit 5**

Agnew, S. M. (1970). The giant sandwich. **Units 3, 2**

Ahlberg (1978). Each peach pear plum. **Unit 2**

Aliki (1994). Christmas tree memories. **Units 3, 5, 2**

Aliki. (1992). Milk from cow to carton. **Unit 2**

Aliki. (1979). The two of them. **Units 5, 3**

Altman, L. J. (1993). Amelia's road. **Units 4, 5, 2**

Aylesworth, J. (1992). The folks in the valley. **Units 5, 4**

Balian, L. (1994). The sweet touch. **Unit 2**

Bang, M. (1984). The grey lady and the strawberry snatcher. **Units 5, 2**

Baron-Hall, D. (1989). Only at the children's table. **Units 2, 3**

Barrett, J. (1986). Pickles have pimples. **Unit 2**

Barrett, J. (1978). Cloudy with a chance of meatballs. **Unit 2**

Bider, D. (1989). A drop of honey. **Units 5, 2, 3**

Bond, R. (1988). Cherry tree. **Units 5, 4, 2**

Breinburg, P. (1974). Doctor shawn. **Unit 3, 5**

Brooks, B. (1991). Lemonade parade. **Units 3, 2**

Brown, M. (1951). Skipper john's cook. **Units 2, 3**

Brown, M. (1947). Stone soup. **Unit 2**

Budd, L. (1960). The pie wagon. **Units 3, 2**

Caines, J. (1988). I need a lunchbox. **Units 3**

Carle, E. (1992). Pancakes, pancakes! **Units 3, 2, 4**

Carle, E. (1993). Today is monday. **Units 3**

Carle, E. (1995). Walter the baker. **Units 3, 2**

Carrick, D. (1985). Milk. **Unit 2**

Choi, S. N. (1993). Halmoni and the picnic. **Units 5, 3**

Cohen, B. (1988). Don't eat too much turkey. **Unit 3**

Cohen, B. (1987). The carp in the bathtub. **Units 5, 2**

Cohen, P. &. L. O. (1989). Olson's meat pies. **Units 3, 2**

Coldrey, J., & Bernard, G. (1988). Strawberry. **Unit 2**

Cole, S. (1991). When the rain stops. **Unit 2**

Creedle, E. (1934). Down down the mountain. **Units 4, 2, 5**

Czernecki, S., & Rhodes, T. (1992). The sleeping bread. **Units 3, 5, 2**

Dalton, A. (1992). This is the way. **Unit 3**

Darling, B. (1992). Valerie and the silver pear. **Units 5, 2, 3**

Day, J. W. (1976). What is a fruit? **Unit 2**

de Bourgoing & Jeunesse, G. (1989). Vegetables in the garden. **Unit 2**

de Regniers, B. S. (1989). May i bring a friend? **Units 2, 3**

de Regniers, B. S. (1987). The snow party. **Units 3, 2**

Degen, B. (1985). Jamberry. **Units 2**

dePaola, T. (1978). Pancakes for breakfast. **Units 3, 2, 4**

dePaola, T. (1978). The popcorn book. **Units 2, 5**

dePaola, T. (1993). Tom. **Units 5, 3**

dePaola, T. (1989). Tony's bread. **Units 2, 3**

dePaola, T. (1974). Watch out for the chicken feet in your soup. **Units 5, 3, 2**

DiSalvo-Ryan, D. (1991). Uncle willie and the soup kitchen. **Units 3, 2**

Dragonwagon, C. (1987). Alligator arrived with apples: A potluck alphabet feast. **Unit 2**

Drucker, M. (1992). Grandma's latkes. **Units 5, 2, 3**

Ehlert, L. (1993). Eating the alphabet: Fruits and vegetables from a to z. **Units 2**

Ehlert, L. (1990). Growing vegetable soup. **Units 2, 4**

Ericsson, J. (1993). No milk! **Unit 2, 4**

Falwell, C. (1993). Feast for 10. **Units 5, 3**

Feder, P. K. (1992). Where does the teacher live? **Unit 3**

Florian, D. (1992). A chef. **Units 3, 2**

Forest, H. (1993). The bakers dozen. **Units 3, 2**

Foster, D. V. (1961). A pocketful of seasons. **Unit 4**

Fowler, A. (1994). Apples of your eye. **Unit 2**

Fowler, A. (1994). Corn-on and off the cob. **Unit 2**

Freidman, I. R. (1984). How my parents learned to eat. **Units 5, 3**

Gage, W. (1976). Squash pie. **Units 2, 4**

Garland, S. (1982). Going shopping. **Unit 3**

Garrison, C. (1976). Flim and flam and the big cheese. **Units 3, 2**

Gibbons, G. (1988). Farming. **Unit 4**

Gibbons, G. (1989). Marge's diner. **Unit 3**

Gilman, P. (1990). Grandma and the pirates. **Units 5, 2**

Giovanni, N. (1968). Knoxville, tennessee. **Units 5, 2**

Goldin, B. D. (1993). Cakes and miracles: A purim tale. **Units 5, 2, 3**

Goldin, B. D. (1988). Just enough is plenty: A hanukkah tale. **Units 5, 2**

Good, E. W. (1994). Fall is here! I love it! **Units 4, 2**

Good, E. W. (1990). It's summertime. **Units 4, 2**

Greenaway, K. (1993). A apple pie. **Units 2**

Greeson, J. (1952). The stingy baker. **Units 3, 2**

Grover, M. (1993). Accidental zucchini. **Unit 2**

Gustafson, S. (1990). Alphabet soup: A feast of letters. **Unit 2**

Hall, Z. (1994). It's pumpkin time! **Units 4, 2**

Hammerstein, O. (1992). A real nice clambake. **Unit 2**

Harper, J. (1993). Jalapeno hal. **Unit 2**

Hennessy, B. G. (1992). Jake baked the cake. **Unit 2**

Hennessy, B. G. (1991). The missing tarts. **Unit 2**

Hennessy, B. G. (1992). School days. **Unit 3**

Hest, A. (1994). The midnight eaters. **Units 5, 2**

Hines, A. G. (1988). Daddy makes the best spaghetti. **Units 3, 2**

Hines, A. G. (1991). The greatest picnic in the world. **Unit 3**

Hines, A. G. (1991). Jackie's lunch box. **Unit 3**

Hoban, R. (1981). The great gum drop. **Unit 2**

Holmes, S. (1994). Alphabet zoo. **Unit 2**

Howard, E. F. (1991). Aunt flossie's hat (and crab cakes later). **Units 5, 2, 3**

Howard, J. R. (1992). When i'm hungry. **Unit 3**

Hudson, W. (1993). I love my family. **Units 5, 3**

Hutchins, P. (1989). Don't forget the bacon. **Units 3, 2**

Ipcar, D. (1976). Hard scrabble harvest. **Units 4, 2**

Jaspersohn, W. (1993). Cookies. **Units 2, 3**

Joosse, B. M. (1987). Jam day. **Units 2, 5, 4**

Kelley, T. (1989). Let's eat. **Units 3, 4**

Kimmelman, L. (1989). Frannie's fruits. **Units 3, 2, 4**

Kindersley, D. (1991). My first look at shopping. **Units 3, 2**

Kindersley, D. (1991). My first look at time. **Unit 3**

King, C. (1994). The vegetables go to bed. **Units 2, 4**

Kovalski, M. (1990). Pizza for breakfast. **Units 3, 2**

Krauss, R. (1989). The carrot seed. **Units 4, 2**

Krockover, G., & Krockover, S. (1978). Uncle bill's ice cream shop. **Units 3, 2**

Kroll, S. (1989). The hokey-pokey man. **Units 5, 3, 2**

Kroll, S. (1991). Howard and gracie's luncheonette. **Unit 3**

Lakin, P. (1994). Don't forget. **Units 3, 5, 2**

Lapp, E. (1983). The blueberry bears. **Unit 2**

Leedy, L. (1994). The edible pyramid: Good eating every day. **Units 2, 3**

LeGuin, U. K. (1992). Fish soup. **Unit 2**

Lember, B. H. (1994). A book of fruit. **Units 2, 4**

Lent, B. (1992). Molasses flood. **Unit 2**

Lessac, F. (1989). Caribbean alphabet. **Unit 5**

Levitin (1980). Nobody stole the pie. **Units 3, 2**

Lobel, A. (1989). On market street. **Unit 3**

Locker, T. (1994). Family farm. **Units 4, 5**

Loomis, C. (1994). In the diner. **Unit 3**

Lottridge, C. (1990). One watermelon seed. **Units 4, 2**

Luenn, N. (1990). Nessa's fish. **Units 5, 2**

MacDonald, E. (1990). Mr. macgregor's breakfast egg. **Units 3, 4**

Mahy, M. (1985). Jam. **Unit 2**

Manushkin, F. (1992). Latkes and applesause. **Units 5, 2**

Manushkin, F. (1995). The matzah that papa brought home. **Units 5, 3, 2**

McCloskey, R. (1976). Blueberries for sal. **Unit 2**

McCloskey, R. (1976). One morning in maine. **Unit 2**

McDonald, M. (1991). A great pumpkin switch. **Units 5, 2**

McDonald, M. (1994). The potato man. **Units 5, 3, 2**

McGovern, A. (1986). Stone soup. **Units 3, 2**

McGrath, B. B. (1994). The m & m counting book. **Unit 2**

McGuire, R. (1994). The orange book. **Unit 2**

McKissack, P. C. (1992). A million fish... more or less. **Units 5, 2**

McMillan, B. (1989). Time to.... **Unit 3**

McMillan, B. (1986). Becca backwards, becca frontwards: A book of concept pairs. **Unit 2**

McMillan, B. (1991). Eating fractions. **Unit 2**

McMillan, B. (1988). Growing colors. **Unit 2**

McNulty, F. (1987). The lady and the spider. **Units 2, 4**

Merriam, E. (1993). 12 ways to get to 11. **Unit 2**

Micucci, C. (1992). The life and the times of the apple. **Units 2, 4**

Mitchell, B., & Sandford, J. (1993). Down buttermilk lane. **Units 5, 3, 4**

Moncure, J. B. (1985). What was it before it was bread? **Unit 2**

Moncure, J. B. (1985). What was it before it was orange juice? **Unit 2**

Morris, A. (1989). Bread, bread, bread. **Units 2, 5**

Munz, E. (1975). Happily appley. **Unit 2**

Myers, B. (1990). It happens to everyone. **Unit 3**

Nerlove, M. (1989). Passover. **Units 5, 3**

Newcome, Z. (1991). Rosie goes shopping. **Units 3, 2**

Nikola-Lisa, W. (1991). 1,2,3 thanksgiving. **Units 3, 2**

Nixon, J. L. (1986). Beats me, claude. **Unit 2**

Noble, T. H. (1984). Apple tree christmas. **Units 4, 2**

Nordgvist, S. (1985). Pancake pie. **Units 4, 2**

Nottridge, R. (1991). Apples. **Unit 2**

Novak, M. (1990). Mr. floop's lunch. **Units 3, 2**

Obligado, L. (1993). The chocolate cow. **Units 5, 2, 4**

Olaleye, I. (1994). Bitter bananas. **Units 5, 2, 3**

Otey, M. (1993). Blue moon soup spoon. **Units 2, 3**

Palmisciano, D. (1989). Garden partners. **Units 5, 4, 2**

Parish, P. (1979). Amelia bedelia helps out. **Unit 2**

Parish, P. (1987). Teach us, amelia bedelia. **Unit 2**

Parish, P. (1964). Thank-you, amelia bedelia. **Unit 2**

Paulsen, G. (1995). The tortilla factory. **Units 4, 5**

Penn, M. (1994). The miracle of the potato latkes. **Units 5, 2**

Pochocki, E. (1993). The mushroom man. **Units 4, 2**

Polacco, P. (1993). The bee tree. **Units 5, 4, 2**

Polacco, P. (1992). Chicken sunday. **Units 5, 2**

Polacco, P. (1988). Rechenka's eggs. **Units 5, 3, 2**

Polacco, P. (1990). Thunder cake. **Units 5, 2**

Priceman, M. (1994). How to make an apple pie and see the world. **Units 5, 2, 4**

Rattigan, J. K. (1993). Dumpling soup. **Units 5, 3, 2**

Reiss, J. J. (1987). Colors. **Unit 2**

Reiss, J. (1982). Numbers. **Unit 2**

Reiss, J. J. (1987). Shapes. **Unit 2**

Rice, E. (1990). At grammy's house. **Units 5, 3, 4**

Richardson (1991). Stephen's feast. **Units 3, 2**

Robins, J. (1988). Addie meets max. **Units 3, 2**

Robinson, F. (1994). Vegetables, vegetables! **Unit 2**

Robinson, F. (1992). We love fruit! **Unit 2**

Rockwell, A. (1994). Apples and pumpkins. **Units 4, 2**

Rockwell, H. (1980). My kitchen. **Units 3, 2**

Rose, A. (1973). How does a czar eat potatoes? **Units 5, 2**

Rylant, C. (1985). The relatives came. **Units 5, 3, 2**

Salt, J., & Hawksley, G. (1990). First words and pictures. **Units 3, 2**

Saunders, S. (1982). Fish fry. **Units 2, 3**

Schaefer, J. J. (1994). Miranda's day to dance. **Units 2, 5**

Scheffler, U. (1990). The giant apple. **Units 4, 2**

Sendak, M. (1986). Chicken soup with rice. **Unit 2**

Sendak, M. (1970). In the night kitchen. **Units 3, 2**

Sendak, M. (1963). Where the wild things are. **Unit 3**

Shelby, A. (1991). Potluck. **Units 3**

Shiefman, V. (1994). Sunday potatoes, monday potatoes. **Unit 2**

Slawson, M. B. (1994). Apple picking time. **Units 4, 2**

Soto, G., & Martinez, E. (1993). Too many tamales. **Units 5, 2, 3**

Speed, T. (1994). Hattie baked a wedding cake. **Unit 2**

Spurr, E. (1991). The biggest birthday cake in the world. **Units 2, 3**

Steele, M. (1989). Anna's garden songs. **Unit 2**

Steffy, J. (1987). The school picnic. **Units 5, 3, 4**

Stock, C. (1990). Christmas time. **Unit 2**

Stock, C. (1991). Easter suprise. **Unit 2**

Stock, C. (1990). Thanksgiving treat. **Units 5, 2**

Titherington, J. (1990). Pumpkin pumpkin. **Units 4, 2**

Tobias, T. (1993). Pot luck. **Units 5, 3**

Turner, D. (1989). Bread. **Unit 2**

Valens, A. (1993). Danilo the fruitman. **Units 5, 3, 2**

Van Leeuwen, J. (1974). Too hot for ice cream. **Units 3, 2**

Van Woerkom, D. (1975). Becky and the bear. **Units 5, 2**

Viorst, J. (1987). Alexander and the terrible, horrible, no good, very bad day. **Units 3, 2**

Viorst, J. (1992). The good-bye book. **Unit 3**

Wagner, K. (1990). Chocolate chip cookies. **Unit 2**

Walton (1983). Tea and whoppers. **Unit 2**

Watson, P., & Watson, M. (1994). The market lady and the mango tree. **Units 5, 3, 2**

Watson, W. (1992). Hurray for the fourth of july. **Units 3, 2**

Watts, B. (1987). Potato. **Unit 2**

Watts, B. (1989). Tomato. **Unit 2**

Wellington, M. (1992). Mr. cookie baker. **Units 3, 2**

Westcott, N. B. (1988). The lady with the alligator purse. **Unit 2**

Westcott, N. B. (1992). Peanut butter and jelly. **Unit 2**

Weston, M. (1994). Apple juice tea. **Units 5, 3**

Widman, C. (1992). The lemon drop jar. **Unit 2**

Wilder, L. I. (1994). Winter days in the big woods. **Units 4, 2**

Williams, B. (1978). Jeremy isn't hungry. **Units 3, 2**

Williams, J. (1992). Everyday abc. **Unit 2**

Williams, J. (1992). Playtime 123. **Unit 3**

Williams, S. A. (1992). Working cotton. **Units 5, 4, 2**

Williams, V. B. (1991). Cherries and cherry pits. **Units 5, 2**

Wolff, F. (1993). Seven loaves of bread. **Unit 2**

Wood, A. (1987). Heckedy peg. **Unit 3**

Wynot, J. (1990). The mother's day sandwich. **Units 3, 2**

Yorinks, A. (1986). Louis the fish. **Units 3, 2**

Zimelman, N. (1976). I will tell you of peach stone. **Units 5, 2**

Note: Each book may be listed in multiple units. Go to the unit listed first to find a complete bibliographic reference and an abstract for the book. The units listed second or third will have a bibliographic reference only for the book.

Valerie A. Ubbes, PhD, CHES, is an assistant professor of health education at Miami University (Oxford, OH) where she prepares preK-12 teachers to understand how curriculum, instruction, and assessment work together to enhance the teaching and learning of health education. Her scholarship focuses on the design of curricula and technologies, which integrate health-related topics, concepts, and skills across the preK-16 curriculum. As one way to increase time spent on health education in elementary schools, she established the *Children's Picture Book Database at Miami University*, available at http://www.lib.muohio.edu/pictbks. Valerie continues to explore how cognitive skills and behavioral outcomes contribute to health literacy. A Certified Health Education Specialist, she seeks to improve the health and education status of children, youth, and their families through the coordinated school health program model promoted by the U.S. Centers for Disease Control and Prevention.

Diana M. Spillman, PhD, RD, LD, is an associate professor of Dietetics in the Department of Physical Education, Health, and Sport Studies at Miami University. She received her PhD from the University of Kentucky and her training at the Shriner's Center for Crippled Children (Lexington, KY), the Appalachian Hospital Consortium, and Barnes Hospital (St. Louis, MO). Her teaching and scholarly work focus on nutrition across the lifespan. Diana teaches courses in Food and Nutrition for the Elderly, Perinatal and Child Nutrition, and Fact and Fiction in Health and Nutrition. She enjoys food and nutrition, and her favorite time of the day is lunch.

NOTES

NOTES

NOTES

NOTES

NOTES

NOTES

NOTES

NOTES

NOTES

NOTES

NOTES

NOTES